The Natural PHARMACIST™

W9-CAV-365

Inside—Find the Answers to These Questions and More

☑ Can the herb gymnema reduce my need for insulin? (See page 48.)

☑ What other herbs can reduce my need for insulin? (See page 56.)

☑ How can I help control my blood sugar with chromium? (See page 35.)

☑ How can the food spice fenugreek reduce my blood sugar level? (See page 53.)

☑ If I have diabetic nerve pain, how can I use lipoic acid to improve my symptoms? (See page 68.)

☑ Are there certain herbs and nutrients I can take to help prevent cataracts from forming? (See page 98.)

☑ What nutritional deficiencies might my diabetes cause, and what can I do about it? (See page 127.)

☑ Can diabetes be prevented? (See page 138.)

☑ Can I have high blood sugar for years and never know it? (See page xi.)

☑ Why is it so important to keep my blood sugar levels closely regulated? (See page 16.)

THE NATURAL PHARMACIST Library

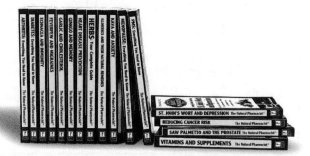

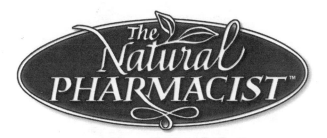

Everything You Need to Know About

Diabetes

Kathi Head, N.D.

Series Editors

Steven Bratman, M.D.

David Kroll, Ph.D.

Prima
HEALTH

A DIVISION OF PRIMA PUBLISHING

Visit us online at www.thenaturalpharmacist.com

This book is dedicated to Peter
and Itty Bitty, the Charismatic Kitty.
You both taught me what it's like to live with diabetes.

Library of Congress Cataloging-in-Publication Data

Head, Kathi
    Diabetes / Kathi Head.
        p.   cm. — (The natural pharmacist)
    Includes bibliographical references and index.
    ISBN 0-7615-1755-3
    1. Diabetes—Popular works.   2. Naturopathy—Popular works.
3. Dietary supplements—Popular works.   4. Herbs—Therapeutic use.
I. Title.   II. Series.
RC660.4.H43 1998
616.4'62—dc21   98-49613
                                                                           CIP

            00 01 02 HH 10 9 8 7 6 5 4 3
            Printed in the United States of America

Visit us online at www.thenaturalpharmacist.com

Contents

What Makes This Book Different?

The interest in natural medicine has never been greater. According to the National Association of Chain Drug Stores, 65 million Americans are using natural supplements, and the number is growing! Yet it is hard for the consumer to find trustworthy sources for balanced information about this emerging field. Why? Frankly, natural medicine has had a checkered history. From snake oil potions sold at the turn of the century to those books, magazines, and product catalogs that hype miracle cures today, this is a field where exaggerated claims have been the norm. Proponents of natural medicine have tended to abuse science, treating it more as a marketing tool than a means of discovering the truth.

But there is truth to be found. Studies of vitamins, minerals, and other food supplements have been with us since these nutritional substances were first discovered, and the level and quality of this science has grown dramatically in the last 20 years. Herbal medicine has been neglected in the United States, but in Europe, this, the oldest of all healing arts, has been the subject of tremendous and ongoing scientific interest.

At present, for a number of herbs and supplements, it is possible to give reasonably scientific answers to the questions: How well does this work? How safe is it? What types of conditions is it best used for?

THE NATURAL PHARMACIST series is designed to cut through the hype and tell you what we know and what we don't know about popular natural treatments. These books are more conservative than any others available, more honest about the weaknesses of natural approaches, more fair in their comparisons of natural and conventional treatments. You won't find any miracle cures here, but you will discover useful options that can help you become healthier.

Why Choose Natural Treatments?

Although the science behind natural medicine continues to grow, this is still a much less scientifically validated field than conventional medicine. You might ask, "Why should I resort to an herb that is only partly proven, when I could take a drug with solid science behind it?" There are at least three good reasons to consider natural alternatives.

First, some herbs and supplements offer benefits that are not matched by any conventional drug. Vitamin E is a good example. It appears to help prevent prostate cancer, a benefit that no standard medication can claim. Also, vitamin E almost certainly helps prevent heart disease. While there are standard drugs that also prevent heart disease, vitamin E works differently and may be able to complement many of the other approaches.

Another example is the herb milk thistle. Studies strongly suggest that this herb can protect the liver from injury. There is no pill or tablet your doctor can prescribe to do the same.

Even if the science behind some of these treatments is less than perfect, when the risks are low and the possible benefit high, a treatment may be worth trying. It is a little-known fact that for many conventional treatments the science is less than perfect as well, and physicians must balance uncertain benefits against incompletely understood risks.

A second reason to consider natural therapies is that some may offer benefits comparable to those of drugs with fewer side effects. The herb St. John's wort is a good example. Reasonably strong scientific evidence suggests that this herb is an effective treatment for mild to moderate depression, while producing fewer side effects on average than conventional medications. Saw palmetto for benign enlargement of the prostate, ginkgo for relieving symptoms and perhaps slowing the progression of Alzheimer's disease, and glucosamine for osteoarthritis are other examples. This is not to say that herbs and supplements are completely harmless—they're not—but for most the level of risk is quite low.

Finally, there is a philosophical point to consider. For many people, it "feels" better to use a treatment that comes from nature instead of from a laboratory. Just as you might rather wear all-cotton clothing than polyester, or look at a mountain landscape rather than the skyscrapers of a downtown city, natural treatments may simply feel more compatible with your view of life. We can quibble endlessly about just what "natural" means and whether a certain treatment is "actually" natural or not, but such arguments are beside the point. The difference is in the feeling, and feelings matter. In fact, having a good feeling about taking an herb may lead you to use it more consistently than you would a prescription drug

Of course, at times synthetic drugs may be necessary and even lifesaving. But on many other occasions it may be quite reasonable to turn to an herb or supplement instead of a drug.

To make good decisions you need good information. Unfortunately, while hundreds of books on alternative medicine are published every year, many are highly misleading. The phrase "studies prove" is often used when the studies in question are so small or so badly conducted that they prove nothing at all. You may even find that the "data" from other books come from studies with petri dishes and not real people!

You can't even assume that books written by well-known authors are scientifically sound. Many of these authors rely on secondary writers, leading to a game of "telephone," where misconceptions are passed around from book to book. And there's a strong tendency to exaggerate the power of natural remedies, whitewashing them with selective reporting.

THE NATURAL PHARMACIST series gives you the balanced information you need to make informed decisions about your health needs. Setting a new, high standard of accuracy and objectivity, these books take a realistic look at the herbs and supplements you read about in the news. You will encounter both favorable and unfavorable studies in these pages and will learn about both the benefits and the risks of natural treatments.

THE NATURAL PHARMACIST series is the source you can trust.

Steven Bratman, M.D.
David Kroll, Ph.D.

Introduction

It is estimated that as many as 16 million Americans are afflicted with diabetes, including as many as 5.4 million people not yet diagnosed. These shocking statistics were reported by the Centers for Disease Control in an article in the Associated Press, June 23, 1998. "Diabetes is the leading cause of adult blindness, end-stage kidney disease and amputations of the foot and leg," reported Dr. James Mark of the CDC. It may go undiagnosed for years, as the onset is often insidious, with few or no symptoms in the early stages. Chronic diseases such as diabetes, heart disease, cancer, and arthritis pose serious threats to both the health and the pocketbooks of the American public. While conventional medicine offers many valuable interventions for such conditions, there is considerably more that can be done, both in the areas of prevention and treatment.

Even with constant monitoring of blood glucose levels and careful administration of insulin or other blood sugar-lowering medications, perfect control of blood sugar is next to impossible, and side effects of high glucose levels eventually develop. Natural medicines can help both control blood sugar levels and prevent the complications of diabetes. The purpose of this book is to share and evaluate the clinical experience and available research on various nutritional supplements, herbs, and dietary approaches for diabetes.

Natural medical approaches can also be helpful in preventing diabetes. While it has long been known that type 2 (non-insulin dependent) diabetes can usually be prevented with diet and lifestyle modifications, exciting new research suggests it may be possible to prevent type 1 (insulin dependent) diabetes as well. The goal of this book is to provide information to both improve the quality and length of life of people with blood sugar problems and help prevent the disease in those who are at risk.

Although alternative medicine has much to offer for the prevention and treatment of diabetes, for a disease as serious as this one it is of utmost importance to continue care with your physician and to inform him or her of the options you are interested in pursuing. Although confiding to your primary doctor that you are also seeking alternative treatment might pose some discomfort, it is absolutely essential in order to avoid potentially serious interactions between drugs and vitamins or herbs.

Never stop medication without guidance from a physician. Keeping blood sugar under control is the primary goal in treating diabetes and, in all cases of type 1 diabetes and some cases of type 2 diabetes, insulin is absolutely required. The goal is to use alternatives to aid in better blood sugar control and prevent complications, NOT TO SUBSTITUTE FOR INSULIN.

The Natural Pharmacist Guide to Diabetes can help people with diabetes or those who have loved ones with diabetes, and those at risk because of family history, obesity, or other factors. Health care practitioners, pharmacists and others who care for and advise people with diabetes can also benefit from the wealth of information contained here.

Diabetes

A Quick Course
in Diabetes

A s a naturopathic physician, I've cared for diabetic patients for many years, using natural remedies to supplement their conventional treatments. Of course I care about all my patients, but I feel particularly connected to those with diabetes because of an incident that happened about a dozen years ago. That's when I had my first "up close and personal" experience with this often devastating illness.

At the time of this incident, I was just starting my practice. My experience with the disease was limited to my clinical knowledge and interactions with patients as a student doctor. One night, however, all that changed, and I received stark and unforgettable insight into what it means to live with diabetes.

I was traveling across the country with my friend Chris, an insulin-dependent diabetic. The trip was great, and he seemed to have his diabetes under control to the extent that I gave it little thought. One night, we checked into a motel near Tucson. As usual, we went for a walk after dinner, then retired to our motel to get ready for bed.

Sometime in the middle of the night, I was awakened by the sound of Chris's thrashing arms and legs hitting the wall in the other room. When I entered his room, I found him in convulsions. Terrified, I realized he must have overestimated how much insulin he needed in his bedtime shot and was now paying the price—life-threatening convulsions brought on by severe low blood sugar. He needed to swallow some sugar to bring his blood sugar back up, but there was no way he could do that in his current condition.

I knew he had to have help fast. My own heart beating wildly, I tried to call 911. Unfortunately, dialing "911" just got me motel room number 911. I tried to call an outside operator by dialing 0, but all that did was wake up the snoozing front desk attendant. There was no way to dial 911 from the motel room!

Half-dressed, half-hysterical, and with one contact lens in, I raced to the motel office. I finally convinced the desk clerk that I had a medical emergency on my hands, and he let me use the phone to call for help. When the paramedics finally arrived, I was shocked to learn they were not equipped to administer intravenous glucose, the sugar he needed to balance his system. I was living a nightmare.

Fortunately, Chris's body's natural safeguards finally kicked in, and his blood sugar returned to normal before any permanent harm occurred. The next morning, we were both emotionally drained but thankful. Chris was in good enough shape to laugh when I told him about dialing 911, and we were soon on our way across country again.

For Chris, the experience was unpleasant and upsetting, but he was philosophical since he had to deal with his diabetes every day. For me, it was an eye-opening glimpse into the difficult life of a diabetic. From that point on, I made it my business to explore all the information I could find on treatments for diabetes, both natural and conventional—anything that could help people with this disease stay healthy and in control of their lives. Since that time I've had personal experiences with other close friends, acquaintances, and even a favorite cat with diabetes.

As a naturopathic physician, I commonly work with diabetics, using natural remedies to supplement the standard treatments of insulin, diet, exercise, and pills. I never forget, though, that those with the most important role in diabetes care are the people who have the disease. Their own knowledge, decisions, and actions have the greatest influence on their health.

If you have diabetes, you undoubtedly know a great deal about this difficult disease. But please bear with me as I present the nuts and bolts of diabetes in this chapter. This information is crucial to your understanding the natural treatments you'll read about later in the book.

What Is Diabetes?

Simply stated, diabetes is a disease that results in excessively high levels of glucose (sugar) in the blood. In some cases, the disease can be silent for years, with the person experiencing few if any symptoms. In other cases, especially when it comes on suddenly, diabetes can lead to unconsciousness and profound derangement of the body's metabolism.

Diabetes is caused by problems with the hormone *insulin.* Here's what happens: Circulating blood always carries a certain amount of glucose (sugar) that provides fuel for the cells. Getting sugar into the cells requires insulin, which is produced in the pancreas by what are called beta cells. Normally, the pancreas produces just enough insulin

What's the Difference Between Type 1 and Type 2 Diabetes?

Type 1:

- *Who gets it:* typically people under the age of 20, although this type can be diagnosed up to about age 40. Many people with type 1 diabetes aren't aware of a family history of the disease.
- *What's going on:* the body attacks the cells that create insulin.
- *Causes:* genetic predisposition combined with exposure to a "trigger," possibly a virus, allergen, or both.
- *Symptoms:* occur weeks to months before diagnosis, and may progress to an emergency situation called diabetic ketoacidosis.

to handle the body's needs from moment to moment. However, in diabetes, insulin is either absent, in short supply, or unable to perform its job effectively.

If glucose cannot get into the cells, it accumulates in the bloodstream, creating high blood sugar. Glucose can also accumulate in certain tissues that don't require insulin for it to enter.

Symptoms of high blood sugar can include excessive thirst, voracious appetite, frequent urination, weight loss, weakness, muscle wasting, and fatigue. If blood sugar levels are allowed to remain excessively high, the person may become comatose. Nonetheless, some people walk around with high blood sugar for years and never know it!

Blood glucose is measured in milligrams per deciliter (mg/dL) of blood. Normally, your blood sugar should be

- *Treatment:* insulin (always required) and careful attention to diet and exercise.

Type 2:

- *Who gets it:* typically overweight people, age 40 and older; there may be a family history of the disease.
- *What's going on:* the body does not respond normally to insulin.
- *Causes:* obesity, heredity, possibly other causes.
- *Symptoms:* may occur for years before diagnosis and can lead to diabetic hyperosmolar coma.
- *Treatment:* diet, exercise, and weight loss; may require oral drugs or insulin.

between about 70 and 110 mg/dL if you're tested when fasting, and up to 130 mg/dL or so after you eat. A person who has a fasting blood sugar of 126 mg/dL or higher on at least two occasions is said to have diabetes. Less commonly, physicians may diagnose diabetes when a blood sugar of 200 mg/dL or higher is measured after eating or during a 2-hour glucose tolerance test. As the value of good blood sugar control in preventing diabetic complications has become more evident, diagnosis guidelines have become stricter. (Before 1997, a fasting blood sugar of 140 mg/dL or higher was considered diagnostic.)

There are two main types of diabetes: type 1, also referred to as insulin dependent diabetes (IDDM) or childhood or juvenile onset diabetes; and type 2, also called non-insulin dependent diabetes (NIDDM) or adult onset

Mark's Story

Mark was a healthy, active 15 year old who loved soccer and science. One Sunday in October, his mother noticed the juice she had bought the day before was gone—two gallons of it. Mark told her he'd been especially thirsty and had drunk it all. He'd also skipped soccer practice because he was too tired. His mother was puzzled, but not worried. A week later, Mark was still drinking and urinating voluminous amounts, and was so tired he wouldn't get out of bed. His mother called the doctor. The next day Mark got his diagnosis: type 1 diabetes.

Because Mark was very interested in natural remedies, at first he hoped he could take some herb that would eliminate

diabetes. (For a quick comparison of the two, see the sidebar entitled What's the Difference Between Type 1 and Type 2 Diabetes?)

What Is Type 1 Diabetes?

In type 1 diabetes, the beta cells of the pancreas become damaged and are ultimately destroyed. When this happens, the pancreas produces very little or no insulin. With this type of diabetes, insulin injections are absolutely necessary.

People with type 1 diabetes comprise only about 5 to 10% of the total number of diabetics in the United States. They are typically diagnosed during childhood or young adulthood. Since even adults in their thirties or older can develop this type of diabetes, the terms "juvenile" and "childhood onset" are not technically correct.

the disease. He was disappointed to learn that no such herb existed. He had to get used to testing his blood sugar and injecting insulin—not just once, but several times a day—in order to prevent complications. The good news he learned was that he could do much to prevent complications by carefully controlling his blood sugar. But he still wondered whether he could use other remedies besides this "standard treatment." His doctor suggested Mark do his own research, and told Mark he'd be glad to work with him in trying any promising herb or supplement options he found. Mark didn't know where to go for reliable information—and unfortunately his doctor didn't know either.

What Causes Type 1 Diabetes?

Although the causes of type 1 diabetes are still being investigated, we do know some things. First, the person must have a genetic predisposition to develop the disease. Only about 5 to 10% of type 1 diabetics have relatives in their immediate family with the same type of diabetes. However, this is a higher percentage than would be expected if no genetic effect existed.

Secondly, heredity alone isn't enough to cause the diabetes. Something in the environment—perhaps a virus or allergen—must trigger the disease. No definite triggers have been identified yet, but some scientists are looking at cow's milk allergy, which I will discuss in chapter 9.

An interesting phone consultation I recently had with a woman on the East Coast seemed to suggest the virus-trigger theory. She told me that her two children had just been diagnosed with diabetes within a week of each other, and the diagnosis came after both had been sick with an upper respiratory virus. Did the virus initiate the diabetes? I don't know. Regardless, my heart went out to her. Having one child with diabetes can be very challenging; coping with two, particularly when they are diagnosed at the same time, can be nearly a full-time job.

How does the trigger for diabetes work? The most widely accepted theory is that the trigger causes the body to treat the beta cells in the pancreas (the cells that produce insulin) as if they were germs. In this situation, called an *autoimmune reaction,* the body produces antibodies against the beta cells. Like heat-seeking missiles, these antibodies seek, attack, and destroy these insulin-producing cells. Eventually, no cells are left to secrete insulin. This process can happen rapidly over a matter of weeks or slowly over months or even years, during which time the person may have no symptoms.

Natural remedies described in this book might help stabilize blood sugar and help prevent or treat some complications of diabetes.

The cells of the body need glucose in order to function normally. In type 1 diabetes, even though the bloodstream contains more than enough circulating glucose, it can't get into the cells due to the lack of insulin. The body tries to get the fuel it needs in other ways, often by breaking down proteins. To do this it tries to digest its own muscles. The result is weight loss, weakness, and muscle wasting.

Even though the disease may have been progressing for a long time, once a critical number of the beta cells are destroyed, the symptoms of type 1 diabetes can come on fast, in a way that's hard to ignore. Generally none of the long-term complications of diabetes have had time to develop by the time the disease is diagnosed.

This book is written for people like Mark, as well as all those with the easier to treat but still serious type 2 diabetes.

How Is Type 1 Diabetes Treated?

If you have type 1 diabetes, you need insulin every day. You also know you must watch what you eat and even how much you exercise, because these can affect the insulin dose you require. But maybe you've wondered whether natural alternatives are available that might help you. The answer? Nothing can replace insulin, diet, and exercise. But some of the natural remedies described in this book might help stabilize blood sugar and help prevent or treat some complications of diabetes. Discussion of natural remedies begins in chapter 3.

What Is Type 2 Diabetes?

Type 2 diabetes, also called non-insulin dependent diabetes, is far more common than type 1. About 90 to 95% of diabetics have type 2. Unlike type 1, type 2 is strongly linked to dietary and lifestyle factors. In fact, an estimated 85% of type 2 diabetics are either obese or have a past history of obesity. Also, unlike type 1, this type of diabetes is not an autoimmune disease.

What Causes Type 2 Diabetes?

Most people with this type of diabetes are diagnosed after the age of 40, although a small number are diagnosed at an earlier age. Type 2 diabetes is much more clearly hereditary than type 1. If one identical twin has type 2

What Is Obesity?

Obesity used to be defined as being more than 20% above an "ideal" body weight for your height, using different tables for men and women. Now the approach to weight guidelines is based on the Body Mass Index or BMI. Why the switch? The BMI correlates more closely with the amount of body fat a person carries. What poses the most risk is the amount of fat, rather than the weight itself.

Although your BMI can be calculated using a formula, you can most easily determine it using table 1. Please note that the BMI is not accurate for young children, pregnant or nursing women, frail elderly people, or very muscular individuals.

If your weight isn't on the table, you can calculate it with the following formula:

1. Multiply your weight, in pounds, by 703.
2. Multiply your height, in inches, by itself (square it).

diabetes, in 90% of cases the other will also.[1] (In type 1 diabetes, the figure is only 35 to 50%.)

Type 2 diabetes tends to be more insidious, and often has few or no symptoms. Once the blood sugars are consistently over 200 mg/dL, patients will usually experience some increased urination, but few have the significant weight loss associated with type 1 diabetes.

Type 2 diabetes is different from type 1 in one basic way: A type 2 diabetic initially produces enough insulin—often too much in fact—but the body has developed resistance to the insulin. Why does this happen?

Our cells have *receptor sites* on their surfaces. These sites are like docking stations that allow specific sub-

3. Divide the first number (weight × 703) by the second number (your height squared).
   That is your BMI.

According to the World Health Organization:

- Ideal body weight is considered to be a BMI between 18.5 and 25.
- Those with a BMI of 25–30 are considered overweight.
- A BMI of 30 or greater is considered obese.

To put this all in perspective in regard to your risk of developing type 2 diabetes:

- A BMI of 27–29 (versus a BMI of 22–23) increases your risk 1,480% (15 times)
- A BMI of 29–31 increases your risk 2,660% (26 times)
- A BMI of 31–33 increases your risk 3,930% (~40 times)
- A BMI of 33–35 increases your risk 5,300% (53 times)

stances to "lock on" and activate processes inside the cells. The more receptor sites on the cell surface, the more efficiently the substance can stimulate cell activity. Obesity can cause the number of receptors for insulin to decrease. Losing weight causes the number of these receptors to increase. Some people with type 2 diabetes have the right number of insulin receptors, but they don't work properly.

Whatever its cause, type 2 diabetes doesn't happen all at once; it develops in stages. Here's a common scenario:

Jan ate a typical American diet high in fat and carbohydrate. She loved chips and burgers, and they ended up on her hips and waist. Because she preferred reading to running, the weight stayed on. Eventually Jan became obese.

Table 1. Weight Guidelines

BMI	21	22	23	24	25	26	27	28	29	30	31
					WEIGHT/POUNDS						
HEIGHT					OVERWEIGHT					OBESE	
5'	107	112	118	123	128	133	138	143	148	153	158
5'1"	111	116	122	127	132	137	143	148	153	158	164
5'2"	115	120	126	131	136	142	147	153	158	164	169
5'3"	118	124	130	135	141	146	152	158	163	169	175
5'4"	122	128	134	140	145	151	157	163	169	174	180
5'5"	126	132	138	144	150	156	162	168	174	180	186
5'6"	130	136	142	148	155	161	167	173	179	186	192
5'7"	134	140	146	153	159	166	172	178	185	191	198
5'8"	138	144	151	158	164	171	177	184	190	197	203
5'9"	142	149	155	162	169	176	182	189	196	203	209
5'10"	146	153	160	167	174	181	188	195	202	209	216
5'11"	150	157	165	172	179	186	193	200	208	215	222
6'	154	162	169	177	184	191	199	206	213	221	228
6'1"	159	166	174	182	189	197	204	212	219	227	234

Adapted from the National Center for Health Statistics.

In response to her weight gain, Jan's body probably made fewer and fewer insulin receptor sites. The few that were left became sluggish. This led to *insulin resistance syndrome:* Her cells no longer responded properly to insulin. In response, Jan's pancreas tried to compensate by pouring more insulin into her body. Her beta cells began to "burn out" under the strain. Jan got a double whammy: insulin resistance and less insulin production. The result was type 2 diabetes.

Because it can take so long to develop, and because the body continues to produce some insulin, type 2 diabetes often goes undiagnosed for years. Often some of the complications of chronically high blood sugar have developed by the time the diagnosis of diabetes is made. Jan was lucky. Savvy to the symptoms of diabetes, she went to the doctor before any complications occurred. And with good blood sugar control, she may avoid complications altogether. She might also consider natural remedies to help prevent complications.

How Is Type 2 Diabetes Treated?

Unlike type 1 diabetes, type 2 does *not* necessarily require insulin injections, because a variety of oral medications can be used. But even better *this disease can usually be controlled by weight loss and lifestyle changes alone.*

If you have type 2 diabetes and are overweight, you may be able to regain normal blood sugar and insulin production just by losing weight. Of course, losing weight isn't always that simple. In this book you will find other natural remedies, in addition to weight loss, that may help control your blood sugar and prevent or treat some of the complications of diabetes.

To read about natural remedies right away, skip to chapter 3.

Acute Complications of Diabetes: Medical Emergencies

Diabetes is a serious condition. Acute complications of diabetes are medical emergencies. Both type 1 and type 2 diabetics can experience life-threatening crises, although they tend to take somewhat different forms as described later.

Ketoacidosis

In type 1 diabetics, excessively high blood sugars may result in a condition called *ketoacidosis*. Ketoacidosis can develop from inadequate doses of insulin. Infection, surgery, or emotional stress can trigger this catastrophic condition.

Ketoacidosis is a condition that occurs when the body uses too much fat as fuel. If the body is able to use glucose as fuel, it will. But diabetics who can't use their glucose will burn their fat, resulting in the production of *ketones*, the breakdown products of fats. Among type 1 diabetics, ketones can accumulate in the blood, upsetting the delicate balance of chemicals and leading to severe dehydration.

People with ketoacidosis develop hyperventilation, weakness, fatigue, abdominal pain, nausea, and vomiting. Their breath may smell like Juicy Fruit gum. They can slide into a "diabetic coma"—an altered state of apathy and stupor. Without treatment, they would die. Today, prompt medical attention to rectify the chemical and sugar imbalance in the blood corrects the problem.

Hyperosmolar Syndrome

Although they don't develop ketoacidosis, type 2 diabetics can experience a different kind of catastrophe, known as hyperosmolar syndrome. High blood sugar causes increased urination and loss of fluid. If the person is taking diuretics, the condition can get worse. If the person cannot drink enough water to make up for the loss, hyperosmolar coma—even more dangerous than ketoacidosis—can result.

This condition is not an uncommon occurrence for elderly diabetics living alone. They may get sick, lose control of their blood sugar, and forget to drink enough water. The blood sugars are typically very high (sometimes as high as 1000 to 2000 mg/dl), but for reasons that aren't entirely clear, there are no ketones in the bloodstream, as would happen in type 1 diabetes. Severe dehydration leads to low blood pressure, loss of consciousness, and eventually deep coma. These people are treated with intravenous fluids and insulin.

Severe Hypoglycemia (Low Blood Sugar)

This complication does not naturally develop with diabetes, but is caused by the power of the treatments if taken in excessive doses. Remember my friend Chris? Severe hypoglycemia, which is what he had, can result from taking more insulin or oral diabetes medication than you need. It occurs most commonly in people who are on insulin. Exercise and certain illnesses may also contribute to its occurrence.

The symptoms of severe hypoglycemia may include disorientation, irritability, tremors, and profuse clammy perspiration. In extreme cases, loss of consciousness and convulsions can occur. Severe hypoglycemia is clearly a medical emergency.

A person who is conscious and able to chew or drink should immediately chew and swallow glucose tablets or some other form of sugar. If the person is unconscious or unable to chew because of convulsions, he or she needs intravenous glucose or an injection of glucagon. (Glucagon is a hormone that has the opposite effect from insulin. It causes the liver to release stored glucose and thus raise blood sugars.)

Chronic Complications of Diabetes: Long-Term Problems

Prior to the discovery of insulin, diabetic ketoacidosis and hyperosmolar coma were the primary causes of death from diabetes. Today, these conditions are relatively easily prevented and treated. Even loose control of blood sugar levels stops most of these catastrophes from occurring.

However, the long-term complications of diabetes have proven much more difficult to eradicate. The good news is that you can dramatically reduce your risk of all the major complications of diabetes by working with your physician to control your blood sugar levels as closely as possible.[2] The problem is that very precise control of blood sugar is necessary for optimum prevention of long-term complications, and such precise control is not always possible, especially for those with type 1 diabetes. Furthermore, in some cases, strict care to keep blood sugar levels low may not even be appropriate (among people with type 1 diabetes with frequent hypoglycemic attacks, for example).

As we shall see in the following chapters, natural treatments may also be able to help prevent or treat many of these complications. I present a summary here of the problems and some of their treatments. Turn to chapters 5, 6, and 7 for more detailed information on lipoic acid, essential fatty acids, vitamin E, and other natural substances that may help.

Circulation Problems, Heart Disease, and Stroke

Chronically high blood sugar can damage large and small blood vessels, accelerating the development of atherosclerosis ("hardening" of the arteries) as well as causing other forms of damage unique to diabetes. Atherosclerosis in turn causes heart attacks, strokes, kidney damage, and loss of circulation in the legs. People who have had diabetes for at least 10 years have twice the prevalence of coronary artery diseases as nondiabetics.

A diabetic can take many steps to reduce the risk of developing atherosclerosis, including keeping good control of blood sugar levels, reducing cholesterol, and lowering blood pressure. Later in this book, I describe some natural approaches that may be useful, such as vitamin E and magnesium.

Nerve Damage

Just as it can affect blood vessels, chronically high blood sugar can damage nerves. People with long-term diabetes may experience pain or numbness in the arms, legs, and especially the feet. This is called *diabetic peripheral neuropathy*. Neuropathy, or nerve damage, can also affect the nerves controlling internal organs and structures. This so-called *autonomic neuropathy* can cause a variety of symptoms and conditions.

The best approach to preventing nerve damage is to keep blood sugar levels under good control.

For example, if diabetes damages the nerves that control the intestines, the person may alternate between constipation and diarrhea. Neuropathy can also affect the heart, causing abnormal rhythms. Some people with long-term diabetes experience balance problems, dizziness, and impotence.

As for all other diabetic complications, the best approach to preventing nerve damage is to keep blood sugar levels under good control. Natural supplements that may be useful in both preventing and treating diabetic neuropathy include lipoic acid, other antioxidants, and essential fatty acids.

Kidney Problems

High blood sugar can also affect the kidneys. Damage to the kidneys related to diabetes is called *diabetic nephropathy*. Diabetes may damage the tiny filtration units in the kidneys, or result in atherosclerosis blocking the important arteries feeding the kidneys. Extensive kidney damage can result in renal failure—the kidneys no longer work—and the patient must have a kidney transplant or be placed on dialysis.

The best ways to prevent this condition are controlling the blood sugar and taking steps to prevent atherosclerosis.

Eye Problems

The eye is frequently damaged by chronically high blood sugar levels. A by-product of glucose, called sorbitol, can build up in the lens of the eye and cause cataracts. In addition, the blood vessels in the retina can become damaged, leading to *diabetic retinopathy,* a leading cause of blindness.

Although we do not know for sure whether any natural treatments can prevent diabetic retinopathy, some intriguing possibilities are discussed in chapter 6, Diabetic Eye Complications.

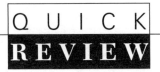

- Diabetes is a disease that results in excessively high levels of glucose (sugar) in the blood. It occurs when the pancreas is unable to produce enough insulin, or when the cells become resistant to insulin, the hormone required to transport glucose into the cells.

- There are two main types of diabetes: type 1 (sometimes called insulin-dependent) and type 2 (sometimes called non-insulin dependent). Type 1 results from a genetic predisposition combined with exposure to an environmental stimulus. Type 2 is strongly linked to heredity and lifestyle factors, both of which can contribute to obesity, dramatically increasing the risk of diabetes.

- Symptoms of diabetes include increased hunger, thirst, frequent urination, weakness, weight loss, and muscle wasting. Type 2 diabetes may present few or no symptoms. The diagnosis of diabetes is based on fasting blood sugar levels of 126 mg/dl or higher, or non-fasting levels of at least 200 mg/dl, each measured on at least two occasions.

- Acute, life-threatening complications of diabetes include severe hypoglycemia, ketoacidosis, and hyperosmolar syndrome. All constitute medical emergencies.

- Chronic complications of high blood sugar can affect the heart and blood vessels, nerves, eyes, and kidneys. Careful blood sugar control can significantly prevent complications, and some natural treatments may help.

Conventional and Dietary Treatment of Diabetes

This book ultimately explores nutritional and herbal approaches you can use to help manage diabetes, but first it's important to review the conventional treatments. While nutritional and herbal approaches may substitute for medications in some diseases, this is definitely not the case in type 1 diabetes (where insulin is necessary), and may not be the case for type 2 diabetes either. These approaches should therefore be regarded as supportive to, rather than replacements for, conventional diabetes management. To understand how to use them, you first need to know something about how conventional medication and dietary therapy for diabetes work. That's what this chapter will cover. If the material is all review for you, then you can skip straight ahead to chapter 3.

Treating Type 1 Diabetes with Insulin

If you have type 1 diabetes, you need daily injections of the hormone insulin. The usual dosage ranges from 30 to

The Development of Insulin

In the late nineteenth and early twentieth centuries, diabetes was poorly understood and commonly fatal. The treatments of choice were "relaxation, massage, opium, and moderate exercise."[1] Children with type 1 diabetes typically died within a year of diagnosis, and people with type 2 suffered far more than they do today.

The discovery of insulin in 1922 was an enormous break-through that gave children with type 1 diabetes their first chance at living to adulthood. The types of insulin available and methods of administration have evolved over the years. They were made originally from pigs and cows. Today's insulin is created in a laboratory. Because it resembles exactly the insulin normally secreted by the human pancreas, it is known as a "human analogue."

---

60 units per day, although this may vary from person to person, and even in the same person from day to day.

Your Needs May Change from Day to Day

A number of factors can influence your daily insulin needs; your stress level, how much exercise you're getting, and what you've eaten all play important roles. Illness— even something as minor as a cold—can dramatically affect the amount of insulin you need to keep your blood sugar in the normal range. Estimating these amounts is not always easy and mistakes can be critical, as Chris's story in chapter 1 illustrated.

What's more, onset of action, duration, and peak activity times of insulin also vary among different people or even within the same person. They depend on the site of

A Quick Guide to Insulin Activity Rates

Insulin lispro (Humalog):
- *Rapid onset:* within 15 minutes
- *Peak effect:* within 1 hour
- *Activity duration:* 2 to 4 hours

Regular:
- *Onset:* within 30 minutes
- *Peak effect:* within 2.5 to 5 hours
- *Activity duration:* 6 to 8 hours

NPH or lente:
- *Onset:* within 1.5 hours for NPH, 2.5 hours for lente
- *Peak effect:* within 4 to 12 hours for NPH, 7 to 15 hours for lente
- *Activity duration:* 18 to 24 hours

injection (for example, thigh or abdomen), level of exercise, and other individual factors.

Finally, the amount of insulin you need to take and when to take it depends not only on the type of insulin injected and your usual response, but also on how high your blood sugar is at the time of injection. For instance, if blood sugar is very high in the morning after testing, the insulin injected must first bring down the already high blood sugar before it can help metabolize breakfast.

How Many Types of Insulin Are There?

We categorize insulin according to the length of time required for the hormone to begin working and the duration of its activity. The most common types of insulin today are fast-acting (regular) and intermediate-acting (NPH and lente). A very fast-acting form, called Humalog (its generic name is insulin lispro), was approved in 1996 and is gaining popularity. Some people with type 1 also take a very long-acting variety.

The types of insulin differ with regard to rate of onset and length of activity because the body absorbs them at different rates. Typically, doctors prescribe a mixture of types. The sidebar, A Quick Guide to Insulin Activity Rates, summarizes the differences between the three basic types of insulin.

Insulin and Blood Sugar Control

Carefully monitoring and controlling your blood sugar levels is the key to avoiding later complications of diabetes. In the past, doctors typically recommended one to two daily injections of insulin for people with type 1 diabetes. Today, however, the goal for people with both types of diabetes is to mimic as closely as possible the way your pancreas would normally secrete insulin. That's why doctors most often prescribe intensive insulin therapy—frequent blood sugar monitoring and several insulin injections every day—for people with type 1. People with type 2 can also apply intensive management, which might include one daily insulin injection or none at all in combination with frequent daily blood sugar monitoring and other treatments.

This is certainly more work for the diabetic or the caregiver, but the rewards down the road may be worth it. Good evidence shows that tight control of blood sugar can minimize the long-term complications of diabetes. In the short term, however, problems may arise since the closer blood sugar levels are kept near normal, the greater the chances of a dangerous hypoglycemic event. If blood sugar tends to be high, hypoglycemia is less likely, because even at insulin's peak action the person's blood sugar is above the danger range—but more likely to cause complications down the road.

This issue will come up in chapters 3 and 4 as well, when we discuss natural treatments that can help lower blood sugar, such as the herb Gymnema and the supplement chromium. When combined with insulin there is the potential that they may work too well and cause hypoglycemia. For this reason, medical supervision is necessary. You may need to revise your insulin dosage when you start natural treatment.

There are also natural treatments that may reduce the complications of diabetes, such as lipoic acid and evening primrose oil (see chapters 5 through 7). But good blood sugar control is still the most important step.

Good evidence shows that tight control of blood sugar can minimize the long-term complications of diabetes.

To achieve really "tight" control of blood sugar, more and more people are using an external insulin pump to deliver a continuous flow of insulin. This pager-sized device is often worn on a belt with a needle inserted into the skin of the abdomen. It delivers a constant trickle of insulin intended to approximate natural levels. Before a meal, when more insulin is required, the person can press the plunger manually to deliver a larger, carefully measured amount. If you have a pump, it is crucial that you monitor your blood glucose levels so you do not develop either hyperglycemia or hypoglycemia.

Treating Type 2 Diabetes with Drugs

Eating the right foods, getting a moderate amount of exercise, and losing excess weight are often enough to control elevated blood sugar in type 2 diabetes. If this approach is not successful, your doctor may recommend oral medications. If the oral medications aren't adequate, you may need insulin as well.

Let's take a look at how these oral medications work.

Sulfonylureas

The most popular oral medications for type 2 diabetes are a class of drugs called sulfonylureas. These drugs work by stimulating the pancreas to produce more insulin and by making the tissues more sensitive to insulin's action.

Quite a few drugs are available in this broad category, with minor differences such as their duration of action. In many cases, sulfonylureas effectively lower blood sugar levels; sometimes, however, they lose their effectiveness with time or may not even work at all.

Amaryl, a relatively new drug in this category introduced in 1995, is also known by the generic name glimepiride. Amaryl docks at different receptor sites on the cell surface than do other drugs in the sulfonylurea class. It also may have less tendency than other sulfonylureas to lose its effectiveness over time.

Other Classes of Drugs

Three other classes of drugs are approved for treatment of type 2 diabetes: the biguanides, the alpha-glucosidase inhibitors, and the thiazolidinediones. Each works in a different way to help lower blood sugar in type 2 diabetes.

The biguanides work by decreasing glucose production in the liver and enhancing glucose uptake by the muscles. Glucophage (metformin) is in this class.

The alpha-glucosidase inhibitor Precose (acarbose) works in the small intestine, by inhibiting enzymes that digest carbohydrates. This slows the absorption of dietary sugars into the bloodstream. Precose is prescribed either alone or in conjunction with other diabetes medications.

The newest class of diabetes drugs, the thiazolidine-diones, was approved in 1997. These drugs—which include Rezulin (troglitazone)—work by improving the action of insulin, and are prescribed either alone or in conjunction with insulin or another oral medications. Both Rezulin and Glucophage are presently being tested on people at high risk for developing type 2 diabetes to determine whether they can help prevent the disease. Unfortunately, Rezulin has been implicated in at least 35 deaths from liver failure. The area of diabetes prevention is very exciting. In later chapters you will read about natural methods for prevention, including large clinical trials that are presently underway.

New Drugs on the Way

As of 1998, the Pharmaceutical Research and Manufacturers of America reported 21 more diabetes-related medications in the pipeline—in the research, clinical testing, or FDA approval processes.

Combination of Oral Drugs and Natural Treatments

Just as with insulin, evidence suggests that some of the natural treatments discussed in chapters 3 and 4, such as chromium and Gymnema, can allow diabetics to cut down on their dosage of oral diabetes medications. By the same token, such combinations can also cause hypoglycemic reactions. Again, supervision by a qualified healthcare professional is essential.

Treating Diabetes with Changes in Diet

All clinicians recognize that dietary factors play a role in the treatment of diabetes; there are, however, different schools of thought concerning which diet is best.

Three basic goals for diet are generally recommended in both type 1 and type 2 diabetes. The first is assisting in good blood sugar control, preventing both highs and lows. A second goal is to keep your blood fats (lipids) low to prevent cardiovascular disease, a major complication of diabetes. A third goal is simply to provide an optimal diet for health and well-being.

Another goal is important for many people with type 2 diabetes: weight loss. Not everyone with type 2 diabetes is overweight, but for those who are, weight loss may "cure" this disease. Losing weight—and keeping it off—will not always make blood sugar normal, but even a drop of 5 to 10% of your initial body weight can make a big difference.

In 1994 the American Diabetes Association (ADA) issued new recommendations that have radically altered how clinicians and nutritionists approach diet management in diabetes. Based on years of research, the ADA did away with the one-size-fits-all "standard diabetic diet" it had advocated for years.

> **Based on years of research, the ADA did away with the one-size-fits-all "standard diabetic diet" it had advocated for years.**

Recognizing that no one diet is ideal for everyone with diabetes, the ADA no longer endorses one particular plan or recommends the same percentages of macronutrients (protein, fats, and carbohydrates) for everyone. A number of meal-planning systems are used in conventional diabetes care settings. One of the most popular is carbohydrate counting: maintaining a relatively constant level of carbohydrates from day to day.

What is the best diet for a person with diabetes? This question has sparked a huge controversy.

Mariah's Story

Not long ago I had the opportunity to meet Laura, the mother of 9-year-old Mariah who was diagnosed last year with diabetes. I want to share her story because I found Laura very inspiring.

Laura always had Mariah on a good, healthy diet. Luckily Mariah had always liked vegetables. But, when her daughter was diagnosed with diabetes, Laura wondered whether she would still be able to follow the same standards and keep her on what she considered to be a healthy diet.

Laura initially decided to focus on controlling Mariah's carbohydrate intake. However, she felt that Mariah was not getting a balanced diet with this approach—she was eating more fat and protein than Laura felt was wise. She began entering the fat, carbohydrate, and protein content of all the food Mariah ate into a program on her computer, along with information about how these foods, alone or in combination, affected Mariah's blood sugar. Now, a year later, she knows what effect every food her daughter eats will have on her blood sugar! Not only that, but Laura has discovered that the

In the last decade, the controversy has heated up between those advocating a higher-carbohydrate diet and those advocating a moderate- or low-carbohydrate diet. At one end of the carbohydrate spectrum, some physicians recommend diets with as much as 70 to 80% carbohydrate. Influenced by nutrition pioneers Dean Ornish and Nathan Pritikin, these physicians prescribe diets low in fat and higher in complex carbohydrates, such as vegetables, whole grains, and water-soluble fiber such as legumes, pectin, and guar gum. Advocates of this high-carbohydrate

diet that best keeps her daughter's blood sugar under control is also the one she always felt was a good diet for Mariah. The diet that resulted is high in vegetables, nuts, and high-quality protein—fish, meat, and chicken. Mariah also eats high-fiber muffins and other breads in moderation.

Laura has learned that good blood sugar control is much more than counting grams of carbohydrate. For instance, 30 g of carbohydrate in the form of bread increases Mariah's insulin requirement more than does 30 g of winter squash. With careful attention to diet, Mariah is able to maintain normal blood sugars on only 3.5 units of insulin daily—and her glycosylated hemoglobin is normal at 5.1! Her mom also gives her some of the nutritional supplements and herbs that will be discussed in the next chapters.

Mariah's story is a good example of how important it is to determine how a particular diet affects you individually and to evaluate the effect of specific foods on blood sugar levels and medication requirements.

approach for people with diabetes believe that if such diets help prevent heart disease, stroke, and cancer among people in general, they should also be healthful for diabetics, who are at high risk for both heart disease and stroke. In addition, the water-soluble fibers help slow the absorption of glucose from the intestines.

At the other end of the spectrum are physicians recommending diets with as little as 10 to 20% carbohydrate. Their focus is on carbohydrate's role in raising blood sugar. Less carbohydrate, they reason, results in less need for insulin—and more stable blood sugars. If blood sugar swings occur, they tend to be much smaller because of the need for less insulin.

To illustrate this controversy, consider three common American breakfast menus: (1) pancakes with syrup and sausage; (2) bacon and eggs; or (3) oatmeal with lowfat milk, a banana, and two pieces of whole-wheat toast with jelly. Which breakfast do you think would be the *least* healthful for a person with diabetes? You'll need to think about at least two things: prevention of cardiovascular disease—a frequent complication of diabetes—as well as daily blood sugar control.

If you picked menu 1 as the worst offender, you're right on target. Few people would argue that pancakes, syrup, and sausage would be the least desirable from a blood sugar and cardiovascular standpoint.

Now, which diet do you think would be the *most* healthful for a person with diabetes? You may think the answer is obvious; yet this is where the controversy lies. Those who advocate a high fiber diet—whole grains, vegetables, and fruits—with fats and animal protein kept to a minimum would choose menu 3: the oatmeal, banana, and toast.

On the other hand, the advocates of the low carbohydrate diet believe the only way to keep blood sugar under good control is to severely limit intake of whole grains, fruits, pasta, breads, and even starchy vegetables. Limiting the carbohydrate intake means increasing the relative amounts of fat and protein. These experts would advocate menu 2, the bacon-and-egg breakfast without toast.

As often happens in science, research is available to support *both* points of view.

Most clinicians tend to recommend diets in the middle of the carbohydrate spectrum for the majority of their patients with diabetes—generally about 40 to 50% carbohydrate.

Be Consistent!

Determining your ideal diet may be a matter of trial and error. Since your goal is to maintain normal blood sugar, you have an excellent tool to get immediate feedback on the effect of what you are eating: blood sugar testing.

If you do make major dietary changes, do so with your doctor's supervision. That way you can keep track of the effect of your new diet on kidney function, blood fats, and long-term blood sugar control.

Here's the bottom line: Some people with diabetes may be able to keep their blood sugar in good control by consuming a good, high-fiber/high-carbohydrate/lowfat diet consisting of whole grains, legumes, vegetables, fruits, and moderate amounts of lowfat protein (fish, soy, chicken, lowfat dairy products). Other people would find that this diet includes too many carbohydrates, leading to out-of-control blood sugars. They might do better on a moderate- or low-carbohydrate diet, eating the same foods but in different proportions.

So what's the answer? Initially, trial and error under your doctor's supervision. But once you've found a diet that seems to be working for you, stick to it. Be consistent in your diet from day to day. *Consistency is probably the most important factor in blood sugar management.*

QUICK REVIEW

- People with type 1 diabetes must treat their diabetes with daily insulin injections. They usually use a combination of types of insulin. These are categorized according to how fast-acting they are: Humalog (very fast-acting), regular (moderately fast-acting), and NPH or lente (intermediate-acting). Some long-acting forms are used as well.

- Conventional treatment of type 2 diabetes includes making changes in diet and exercise, and often using oral medications and/or insulin. Four general classifications of oral medications are prescribed for diabetes: sulfonylureas, biguanides, alpha-glucosidase inhibitors, and thiazolidinediones. They all use different mechanisms to help lower blood sugar.

- The American Diabetes Association makes dietary recommendations for people with diabetes. Until the last decade, the association urged all diabetics to count calories and include a certain number of "exchanges" from the various food groups in each meal. Today the ADA no longer recommends the same approach for every patient. They focus instead on individualizing meal-planning strategies for good blood sugar and cholesterol control, adequate calories to achieve weight goals, and optimum nutrition for good health.

- A controversy is raging among nutritionally oriented physicians as to the optimum diet for a person with diabetes. On one end of the spectrum are those advocating a high complex carbohydrate/fiber diet; at the other end are those advocating a very low carbohydrate diet. There is evidence to support both points of view.

- The most important aspect of diet is to be consistent and to be aware of the effect each food or combination of foods has on your blood sugar.

Nutrients for the Control of Blood Sugar

Y ou may have heard about chromium, a nutrient that may help control blood sugar. Have you wondered whether any scientific evidence supports its use? In this chapter I will review the scientific literature on chromium, as well as some of the challenges scientists face in studying this fascinating mineral. I'll also discuss some other nutrients that might impact blood sugar—in some cases improving, and in others worsening control. Generally, these nutrients seem most effective when used in high doses—beyond dosages needed to correct nutritional deficiencies.

Before discussing the nutrients, I want to share a few thoughts about research in general since much of the information in this book comes from scientific studies, which can vary greatly in quality. You'll need to know how to determine whether the study is reliable before you can accept or reject its results. A little explanation up front will help you put the information in the rest of the book in perspective.

A Word About Studies

When you read about studies, keep some basic facts in mind. First, the larger the study, the better the base of information. Studies with fewer participants are less likely to yield accurate results than those with a larger number of participants. The people being studied may be somewhat atypical, and their experiences may not reflect what is representative for the general population as well as a larger test group would. The more people studied, the more likely they are to reflect all people who have the condition.

Second, double-blind studies are preferable to other types of studies. In double-blind studies, neither the doctors nor the patients know who is receiving the test treatment, and who is receiving a fake treatment called a "placebo." Sometimes people get well because they *think* they are supposed to get well, not necessarily because the substance being tested really works. This is called the "placebo effect." Can the placebo effect improve blood sugar levels? Probably not very much, but blinded trials are still preferable.

Third, good studies are "controlled." In a controlled study some participants are given the treatment and others—the "control" group—are left untreated or are given a placebo. "Uncontrolled" studies, in which everyone is given the treatment, are highly unreliable because individuals who know they are being treated may naturally begin to pay more attention to their disease and take better care of themselves.

When scientists are just beginning to look at a substance, they may use a less-than-perfect study technique to see whether a larger, more expensive study is worthwhile. Many studies presented in this chapter are of this preliminary type. They may not be controlled or double-blinded, or may include a small number of participants.

Chromium

Chromium, an essential trace mineral, is required for sugar and fat metabolism.[1] Compared to iron and some other nutrients, it's a newcomer to nutritional science. Science didn't establish a role for chromium in the body until 1959. That's when researchers discovered people on hospital tube feedings, who received no chromium whatsoever, developed diabetes.

However, difficulties arose when scientists tried to determine exactly how much chromium is needed. We appear to need only very tiny amounts—typical recommendations range from 50 to 200 micrograms (mcg) daily. One microgram is just 1/1000th of a milligram—a minuscule amount indeed, compared to our needs for other nutrients like protein.

Because of problems measuring this tiny but essential nutrient, chromium still had no recommended dietary allowance (RDA) as of 1998. Despite this uncertainty, studies of people's diets suggest that many of us may be at least somewhat deficient in chromium. Most diets contain less than 30 mcg.[2] The best dietary source is brewer's yeast, not a common item on most people's tables. If you are diabetic, low intake of chromium may be complicated by poor absorption in your digestive tract. If this is the case, you may need to consume more than the average amount to supply your chromium requirement.[3]

Many people may be slightly deficient in chromium for a number of good reasons. You can actually deplete chromium levels in your body by eating a diet high in refined sugar and white flour products. These foods are not only low in chromium, but trigger further chromium loss. Good high-chromium foods include liver, brown rice, cheese, meat, potatoes, whole-wheat bread, and—of course—brewer's yeast.

How Does Chromium Work?

We don't fully understand just how chromium improves blood sugar metabolism. Remember our discussion of cell receptor sites for insulin from chapter 1? Chromium may work partly by helping insulin bind to those receptor sites. At any rate, it appears to decrease insulin resistance and enhance cells' sensitivity to insulin.

Here's an interesting pair of facts: A chromium deficiency results in an increased need for insulin. And excess insulin, such as is seen in many cases of type 2 diabetes, can in turn cause a chromium deficiency. The bottom line is that chromium may be useful for both type 1 and type 2 diabetes.

What Is the Scientific Evidence for Chromium?

Researchers have conducted several human studies on the use of chromium in diabetes (see A Word About Studies). In one 4-month, double-blind study reported in 1997, 180 people with type 2 diabetes were divided into three groups: One group received 100 mcg of chromium twice daily; the second group got 500 mcg chromium twice daily; and the third group got a placebo—a substance that has no effect on diabetes. All participants continued to follow their usual treatments.[4]

The group taking 500 mcg twice daily significantly lowered their fasting blood sugar levels while the other two groups did not. But the most dramatic change came in something called glycosylated hemoglobin, a measure of long-term blood sugar control (see the sidebar, How Well Has Your Blood Sugar Been Controlled in the Past?).

After 4 months, both groups receiving chromium had a significant drop in their glycosylated hemoglobin. The level was down to normal in the group getting the higher dose, unchanged in the group that received the placebo, and in between for the group getting the lower dose. After

4 months, the cholesterol levels were also significantly decreased in the higher dose chromium group.

The researchers concluded that "the beneficial effects of chromium in individuals with diabetes were observed at levels higher than the upper limit" of estimated daily requirements. In a sense, this treatment uses chromium as a drug, though a natural drug.

Scientists are almost never satisfied with one study—they know too well that studies, when repeated, can produce contradictory results. So let's look at several earlier studies to see what results were found.

Another study also showed that chromium helped control blood sugar. In a 1993 study, 243 diabetics took 200 mcg/day of chromium.[5] These patients were aware of the fact they were taking chromium and were told to decrease their oral hypoglycemic medication or insulin as needed in order to avoid hypoglycemic episodes. More than half the people with type 2 diabetes, and more than one-third of those with type 1, were able to cut back on their medications. Notice that study participants did not go off their other glucose-lowering treatments; they simply decreased the amounts they used. This reminder is for those of you who choose to take chromium supplements: Make sure you work closely with your physician to avoid hypoglycemic episodes. Similar results have been seen in other studies.[6, 7]

> **Chromium deficiency causes an increased need for insulin. And the excess insulin that can occur in type 2 diabetes may in turn cause a chromium deficiency.**

How Well Has Your Blood Sugar Been Controlled in the Past?

Have you ever wondered how well you are controlling your blood sugar? The glycosylated hemoglobin, or HbA1c, test estimates how well your blood sugar has been controlled in the recent past.

When blood sugar is high, extra glucose becomes attached to various proteins, including hemoglobin, the oxygen-carrying protein in red blood cells. A protein with glucose attached is said to be "glycosylated," and glycosylated hemoglobin is

All this evidence certainly looks persuasive. However, chromium did not seem to improve blood sugar control in all studies.[8, 9] Why? In one case the dose of chromium was too low. It's not clear what caused the negative result in the other study.

Such contradictions are a common occurrence, even in studies of drugs. In the case of chromium, the balance of the evidence appears to suggest that supplementation can be helpful.

Dosage

If you do decide to try chromium supplementation, talk with your doctor. You may want to review the studies discussed here with him or her to see whether chromium seems a good option for you. The effectiveness of chromium is likely to depend on how much you take. Doses of 50 to 100 mcg daily, although high enough to correct a deficiency, may not be effective at improving blood sugar control. In at least one study, 1,000 mcg daily was found to be more effective than 200 mcg daily. This dose is on the high side, however, and may present safety concerns (see the next section).

called HbA1c. If the test shows that more than about 6.5% of the hemoglobin is glycosylated, the results suggest inadequate average glucose control over the past 3 months or so. Some labs differ in what they consider "normal."

As described in this chapter, one double-blind study reported that chromium supplementation lowered HbA1c levels, indicating that it improved long-term blood sugar control.

Chromium is available in a number of forms, some of which are better absorbed than others. Chromium citrate and picolinate are well absorbed, while chromium chloride is not.

Safety Issues

The Estimated Safe and Adequate Daily Dietary Intake (ESADDI) of chromium has been established at 200 mcg/day by a government agency. However, animal studies have found no toxicity even at oral dosages over 5,000 times this amount. The reference range established by the U.S. Environmental Protection Agency for toxic exposure to chromium is 350 times higher than the ESADDI of 200 mcg.[10] However, a few recent reports suggest that chromium can cause adverse reactions at doses that are excessive, but not that excessive. For example, a woman taking 1,200 to 2,400 mcg of chromium picolinate daily for 4 to 5 months developed anemia, reduction in platelets, weight loss, and liver and kidney toxicity.[11] Kidney problems were reported in a similar case as well.[12]

It is probably reasonable to conclude from all this information that dosages from 200 to 600 mcg daily are safe.

Anya's Story

A few years ago, an Israeli woman named Anya came to my office to discuss her type 2 diabetes. The blood sugar–lowering medication her medical doctor was prescribing had stopped working. Her doctor had suggested a dietary approach instead. She had tried to change her diet, eating fewer desserts and less bread, but her blood sugar was still often over 200 when she checked it. Having read about vanadyl sulfate in a popular holistic newsletter, she wanted to try it.

At the time, I had not read much research on vanadium and did not feel comfortable prescribing the high doses (50 mg twice daily) that were being touted in the newsletter article. I told her we could try lower doses (5 mg twice daily) along with chromium (200 mcg with each meal) and some herbs for

If you wish to try the higher dose of 1,000 mcg daily used in the study described above, make sure your physician is supervising. In any case, you should work with your physician to carefully monitor glucose levels at any dose of chromium, as you should with any supplement that has the potential to lower blood sugar.

The maximum safe dose of chromium in young children, pregnant or nursing women, or people with severe liver or kidney disease has not been established.

Other Supplements That May Help Lower Blood Sugar

Researchers are investigating several other supplements for their possible effectiveness in lowering blood sugar.

lowering blood sugar (see chapter 4). Anya agreed to keep a daily log of her blood sugar levels.

When Anya returned about 6 weeks later she showed me her blood sugar log. Her blood sugar was 180 or below in most cases. Although still somewhat high, it was generally lower than it had been on her first visit. We agreed on some stricter dietary measures and decided to check her glycosylated hemoglobin after she had been on the program for 3 months. Unfortunately, she returned to Israel before she had a chance to come in for a second follow-up visit.

It's hard to say whether the low dose of vanadyl sulfate had any effect, since it was combined with other blood sugar–lowering nutrients and herbs, as well as dietary changes. However, the overall program seemed to offer some benefit.

These include vanadium, biotin, and magnesium. At present, we don't have sufficient evidence to be sure they're helpful, but I'm including the information to inform you of upcoming possibilities for treatment.

Vanadium

Vanadium is a trace mineral that has not been established as an essential nutrient in human nutrition. At the end of the nineteenth century, 20 or 30 years before the discovery of insulin, vanadium (in the form of sodium metavanadate) was used to treat diabetes.[13] Animal studies[14, 15, 16] and a few tiny studies on human type 2 diabetics,[17, 18] point to the possible effectiveness of oral vanadium (in the form of vanadyl sulfate) in controlling blood sugar. More research is clearly needed.

Vanadyl sulfate, which has less potential toxicity than other forms of vanadium, is the form used in recent studies. Because the dosage in the studies, sometimes 100 mg daily, is very high, use of vanadium for the control of blood sugar should be tried only under the care of a physician well trained in nutrition. Incidentally, vanadium has been reported to aggravate manic depression in people with that condition.

Biotin

Biotin, a member of the B-complex family of vitamins, is important for the metabolism of carbohydrates, fats, and proteins. A deficiency of this vitamin is rare because it can be produced by bacteria in the intestines. Preliminary evidence suggests that biotin may be important in diabetes. It appears to improve insulin sensitivity and stimulate an enzyme called glucokinase, which is involved in utilization of glucose in the liver.

In several animal studies, biotin has been found to improve blood sugar metabolism in both type 1 and type 2 diabetic animals, by decreasing glucose levels after a meal, and improving insulin response.[19, 20]

Fewer clinical trials have been performed on the use of biotin for controlling blood sugar in diabetes. In two very short-term placebo-controlled trials, type 1 and 2 diabetic patients experienced a drop in blood sugar when on biotin, in contrast to people in the control group.[21, 22] Researchers, however, have found that diabetics have higher levels of biotin in their bodies than do nondiabetics. Supplementing with high doses is therefore not correcting a deficiency, but may be overcoming some defect in biotin metabolism.

Biotin is generally found in microgram dosages in multiple vitamins, in the range of 300 mcg or so. However, therapeutic dosages for lowering blood sugar may be much higher, in the range of 8 to 16 mg daily.

Biotin is found in high amounts in cooked egg yolk, saltwater fish, meat, poultry, dairy, soybeans, and yeast. Eating raw egg whites or using sulfa drugs and antibiotics can cause a biotin deficiency.

As a water-soluble vitamin that does not appear to accumulate in tissues of the body, toxicity with biotin is unlikely, although pregnant and nursing mothers should avoid high doses.

Niacin

Niacin is contained in many enzymes that are important for carbohydrate metabolism. So it's not surprising that researchers have looked at its use in diabetes. As you will see in chapter 9, a form of niacin called niacinamide may help prevent type 1 diabetes by protecting the insulin-secreting beta cells in the pancreas from destruction. Niacin may also help control blood sugar in some cases, although no strong evidence supports this. In one small case report, four patients with type 2 diabetes were supplemented with niacin at a dose of 500 mg daily for 1 month, followed by 250 mg daily. Blood sugar levels became normal and two of the four patients were able to discontinue their oral medications.[23]

While interesting, a study of this size is not nearly sufficient evidence to prove niacin works. Of more importance may be the possibility that high doses of niacin may actually interfere with blood sugar control (see later).

Magnesium

As I will discuss in chapter 8, diabetics are commonly deficient in magnesium. Researchers have proposed that magnesium within the cell enhances the effects of insulin.[24] One study focused on the effects of high doses of magnesium on older people with type 2 diabetes. In this very small double-blind study, eight people received either 2 g daily of magnesium (in addition to what was in the diet) or placebo for 4 weeks, with 2 weeks in between to "wash" the treatment out of their system.[25] Their glucose metabolism did not change during the placebo period, but both their insulin sensitivity and glucose uptake improved significantly during the time they took magnesium. This dose of magnesium is high enough to have a laxative effect on a large percentage of patients. In addition, high dose magnesium should be avoided in those with kidney disease. A more typical dose for magnesium is in the range of 500 mg daily.

Nutrients That May Impair Glucose Control

A few nutrients—niacin, zinc, and iron—can actually impair blood sugar control in people with diabetes when taken in large doses. Small amounts, on the other hand, may be beneficial. You should be aware of these, particularly if you are taking a variety of supplements.

Niacin

At dosages of 1 to 4 g daily, which are sometimes used to lower cholesterol, niacin may impair glucose tolerance.[26] In addition, this dosage can result in liver toxicity, as well as acute symptoms of flushing, burning skin, and gastrointestinal upset.

Zinc

Some diabetics have been found to be low in zinc, and a deficiency has been related to a decreased response to insulin.[27] However, in at least two studies, zinc supplementation was found to impair glucose metabolism.

In one study, type 1 diabetics receiving 50 mg zinc daily for 28 days demonstrated marked increases in glycosylated hemoglobin.[28] In another small study, of type 2 diabetics, supplementation of 220 mg zinc sulfate (90 mg actual zinc) 3 times daily for 2 months increased fasting glucose from an average of 177 mg/dL to 207 mg/dL.[29] Based on these results, if you are diabetic and want to take significantly more than the RDA of 15 mg zinc daily, you would be wise to monitor your blood sugar levels carefully.

A few nutrients— niacin, zinc, and iron—can actually impair blood sugar control in people with diabetes when taken in large doses.

Iron

Iron is another mineral that may occasionally cause problems with blood sugar. Rather than supplementing with iron, _reducing_ iron levels might improve blood sugar control. In a study of eighteen type 2 diabetics with relatively high blood sugar, nine (50%) were found to have elevated serum ferritin levels (the form of iron stored in the body).[30] In eight of the nine patients with elevated iron stores, taking an iron-chelating drug (a drug to lower iron levels) resulted in significant lowering of blood sugar, glycosylated hemoglobin, cholesterol, and triglycerides. The reduction was permanent and these people were able to discontinue medication.

It appears that for a small subset of diabetics, the cause of the blood sugar abnormality may be elevated iron levels. When these levels are restored to normal, the condition is reversed. Your doctor should check your iron levels—especially if you have type 2 diabetes. Iron supplementation should probably be avoided unless you are definitely low.

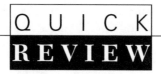

- Of all nutrients, chromium has the most evidence for its effectiveness in controlling blood sugar. It may be useful for both type 1 and type 2 diabetes.

- Because of safety concerns at the higher dosing range, as well as the potential for hypoglycemic episodes if it works too well, close medical supervision is essential when taking chromium.

- Vanadium, biotin, and magnesium may hold promise for lowering blood sugar, but much more research is needed.

- Zinc, iron, and niacin may actually interfere with glucose control.

- When you supplement a nutrient that has the potential of lowering or raising blood sugar levels, careful monitoring is essential.

- When you introduce a nutrient at high dosages, do so only under supervision of a physician who is experienced in nutrition.

Herbal Remedies That May Help Control Blood Sugar

You now know about some nutrients that may lower blood sugar, including chromium. But can any herbs do the same? The answer seems to be yes. Gymnema, bitter melon, and other plant substances have been shown to lower blood sugar in several studies. Not all the studies have been of high quality, and none suggest that these substances will replace insulin for someone with type 1 diabetes. You may, however, find that one or another remedy will improve your blood sugar control or even perhaps reduce your need for medication.

Warning: If you use one of these remedies and it proves effective, *your blood sugar levels will fall.* If you have diabetes, and begin taking any herb or supplement that has the potential of lowering blood sugar, *monitoring is absolutely necessary. Always* let your doctor know what you plan to do and do so under medical supervision. *Do not* simply stop your conventional treatment and treat yourself with herbs! Both type 1 and type 2 diabetics should seek medical advice before changing the dose of any prescription medication.

Ayurvedic (Indian) and Chinese Herbs for Blood Sugar Control

The herbs we'll look at in this section have been used for thousands of years in Ayurvedic medicine in India, or in traditional Chinese medicine. Preliminary studies focusing on several of these plants show promise in treating diabetes. Not surprisingly, many of the studies were conducted in India. Typical dosages are listed in table 2.

Gymnema, bitter melon, and other plant substances have been shown to lower blood sugar in several studies.

None of these herbs have been as extensively studied as, for example, St. John's wort for depression or saw palmetto for prostate enlargement. See A Word About Studies in the previous chapter and keep these points in mind as you read.

Gymnema sylvestre

Gymnema sylvestre is a woody, climbing plant native to India. The leaves of this plant have been used in India for over 2,000 years to treat *madhu meha* or "honey urine" (a traditional name for diabetes). Chewing the plant also destroys the ability to taste "sweet," resulting in its common Indian name: *gur-mar* (sugar-destroyer).

What Is the Scientific Evidence for Gymnema?

Given its long history of use treating diabetes in India, Gymnema has been the subject of considerable animal and human research since the 1930s. Some promising preliminary studies on the use of Gymnema for diabetes, both type 1 and 2, have been conducted. Unfortunately, an extensive search of the literature did not uncover any double-blind studies on this very promising herbal treatment for diabetes.

In one controlled but not blinded study, an extract of the plant was given to 27 type 1 diabetics at a dose of 400 mg/day for 6 to 30 months.[1] Thirty-seven patients continued conventional insulin therapy alone. Among those taking the herb, insulin requirements were decreased by about half. Not only that, but study participants' average blood sugar was reduced from 232 mg/dl to 152 mg/dl. In addition, they had a statistically significant reduction in their glycosylated hemoglobin (HbA1c) after 6 to 8 months on the Gymnema extract, in contrast to the control group, which showed no significant decrease in blood sugar.

Some of this improvement may have been due to the "placebo effect." Although placebo treatments are more likely to influence subjective symptoms such as headaches and pain, they certainly can affect objective measurements as well. However, the changes in blood sugar and glycosylated hemoglobin measured in participants who took Gymnema in this study seem too large to attribute entirely to the placebo effect.

Some of the same researchers conducted a study on people with type 2 diabetes.[2] For 18 to 20 months, Gymnema extract was administered at a dose of 400 mg daily to 22 type 2 diabetics, along with their oral blood sugar–lowering medications. This group experienced significant lowering of blood sugar and glycosylated hemoglobin, and their pancreatic release of insulin increased. The group was able to decrease the dosage of medication, and 5 of the 22 actually were able to discontinue their prescription blood sugar–lowering drugs.

Clearly further research needs to be performed, particularly double-blind studies involving at least 50 people with diabetes (300 or more would be even better).

How Does Gymnema Work?

We don't completely understand how Gymnema may lower blood sugar in humans, but animal studies give us interesting information.

In two studies, researchers gave Gymnema extracts for 1 or 2 months to rats that had been given toxic substances to induce diabetes.[3, 4] The number of insulin-secreting beta cells in the rats doubled, and their insulin levels increased to almost normal. This suggests that Gymnema stimulates regeneration of important insulin-secreting cells in the pancreas. Studies on diabetic rabbits suggest that Gymnema also helps sugar get into the cells.[5]

Further studies have revealed evidence that some of the substances in Gymnema inhibit the absorption of glucose in the intestines.[6] Several mechanisms might work together.

Dosage

Gymnema is sold in a concentrated extract standardized to contain 24% gymnemic acid. The typical dose is 400 to 600 mg daily.

Safety Issues

Side effects are infrequent and there are no reports of severe adverse reactions. Nonetheless, researchers have not yet performed full safety studies; specifically, they have not established the safety of Gymnema for pregnant or nursing women, or for people with severe liver or kidney disease. Also, as for all treatments used to help control blood sugar, the potential clearly exists for excessive lowering of blood sugar. For this reason, medical supervision is strongly advisable when you use this herb.

Momordica charantia

Also known as bitter melon, balsam pear, or bitter gourd, *Momordica charantia* grows in China, India, and Africa. The herb has a long history of use as both food and medicine, particularly in China. Scientists believe the active blood sugar–lowering components of the plant are contained in the fruit and seeds, and include a substance called charantin and an interesting molecule with several aliases: p-insulin, polypeptide-p, or plant insulin.

Bitter melon is available in Asian grocery stores and in herbal formulas sold in pharmacies and health food stores, or is prescribed by alternative medical practitioners.

What Is the Scientific Evidence for Momordica?

P-insulin is a large molecule closely resembling insulin from cows (bovine insulin) in structure and function.[7] When injected under the skin of nine type 1 diabetics, it behaved very much like bovine insulin in terms of the timing of its onset and peak action.[8]

Unfortunately, a search of the literature failed to disclose any published *double-blind* studies on the use of Momordica.

An uncontrolled study was conducted on 18 newly diagnosed type 2 diabetics.[9] Each was given 100 ml of fresh juice from the plant's fruit. This led to significant lowering of blood sugar in 73% of the group, and no change in the other 27%. In another study, five type 2 diabetics were given 15 g per day of the dried powder, while 7 were administered 100 ml of the water extract.[10] Results came in two stages: After 3 weeks, those receiving the dried powder experienced an average blood sugar drop of 25%, while those receiving the liquid extract had an average drop in blood sugar of 54%. After 7 weeks, the liquid-extract group also experienced a significant drop in glycosylated hemoglobin, a measure of long-term glucose control.

Daniel's Story

While attending a health conference in New Orleans recently, I spent some time talking with a man with type 1 diabetes I shall call Daniel, who is also a healthcare professional. After hearing his story, I suggested he try an herbal combination containing Momordica, Gymnema, and chromium. He e-mailed me 2 weeks later to tell me that he had been having low blood sugar episodes since starting to take the formula and, as a result, had lowered his daily insulin dosage from an average of 55 units daily to 42 units daily.

This story exemplifies not only the power of herbs and other supplements to lower blood sugar, but also the importance of careful blood sugar monitoring and physician guidance when introducing new supplements to your treatment plan.

Other studies have found that other forms of Momordica, including whole cooked fruit, can also affect blood sugar.[11, 12]

How Does Momordica Work?

The many animal studies that have found Momordica to lower blood sugar have shed some light on how it works. The decrease in blood sugar appears due—at least in part—to effects outside the pancreas, including increased glucose uptake by cells.[13, 14]

Dosage

The recommended dosage of Momordica depends on the form being consumed. Typical dosage of the fresh juice is within the range of 50 to 100 ml daily, but let me warn you right now: it is incredibly bitter. Capsulized dried powdered fruit is a lot easier to take. The standard dosage is 3 to 15 g daily, which is quite a large dose since the most that can be crammed into a single capsule is about 1 g. Perhaps the best form (because you don't need so much) is a standardized extract. This form should be taken according to the directions on the label, generally in the range of 100 to 200 mg 3 times daily.

Safety Issues

Although Momordica has not been subjected to formal safety studies, its wide use as an Asian food suggests that it is safe. (In some Asian cultures, the fried fruit is eaten daily.) However, safety has not been established in young children, pregnant or nursing women, or those with severe kidney or liver disease.

Fenugreek (*Trigonella foenum graecum*)

Trigonella foenum graecum, commonly known as fenugreek, has been used in India for centuries, both as a medicine and as a condiment in cooking. People with diabetes may find it a useful addition to their diet and treatment. There is evidence that seeds or the defatted seed powder have blood sugar–lowering capabilities in animals, as well as in humans with either type 1 or type 2 diabetes. The fiber portion of the seed appears to contain the active component.[15]

What Is the Scientific Evidence for Fenugreek?

In a controlled study, 10 type 1 diabetics were randomly prescribed either defatted fenugreek seed powder at a dose of 50 g twice daily as part of their lunch and dinner, or the same meals without the powder, each for 10 days.[16] Those on the fenugreek diet had significant decreases in their fasting blood sugar and in urinary glucose.

Melissa's Story

Melissa, an artist with type 2 diabetes, had been taking dried powdered Momordica for several months under the supervision of her naturopathic physician. This treatment had allowed her to reduce the dosage of her standard oral diabetes medication. However, when she traveled out of state to show her work at a national exhibition, she discovered she was nearly out of the remedy. Unworried, she stopped at a pharmacy to see whether she could stock up. Unfortunately they

Double-blind studies have found benefits from lower doses of fenugreek as well. In one study, 21 type 2 diabetics were given a dose of 15 g daily;[17] in a second study 60 people with diabetes took 25 g daily.[18] Significant improvements in blood sugar control, blood sugar elevations in response to a meal, urinary glucose, and even cholesterol were noted.

Numerous studies on dogs, rats, and mice support the potential benefit of fenugreek on blood sugar control. In one study, an alcohol extract of fenugreek seeds given to diabetic mice had an effect comparable to the oral medication tolbutamide.[19]

How Does Fenugreek Work?

According to animal studies, fenugreek may work much the same way as the alpha-glucosidase inhibitor group of drugs discussed in chapter 2, lowering blood sugar by interfering with the intestinal absorption of glucose.[20] However, there is much we do not yet know.

Dosage

A look at the studies involving fenugreek shows a wide range of therapeutic dosage—from 15 to 100 g daily. The

didn't have her brand. The one they did carry looked fine, but she decided to show her old bottle to the pharmacist.

It was lucky she did because the pharmacist pointed out that his stock was a powdered concentrated extract, while Melissa's was the simple dried powder. The two doses were entirely different. Melissa might have sent her blood sugar plummeting had she taken the same dose of the concentrated product as she normally took of the unconcentrated version. Melissa followed the label instructions and did fine.

study of type 1 diabetics used a considerably higher dose (50 g twice daily) compared to the two cited on type 2 diabetics (15 g and 25 g daily). (For dosage recommendations see table 2.)

Taking that much fenugreek in capsule form isn't practical—you would be swallowing pills nonstop. A more reasonable approach is to mix the powder in food or water and incorporate it into the meal. Unfortunately, the dried herb alone doesn't have the desired effects, but you can cook with the defatted seed powder. The mother of the two children with diabetes—the kids diagnosed within a week of each other—uses it in baking. To give you an idea of how much we're talking about, one slightly rounded tablespoon of defatted fenugreek powder weighs about 10.5 g.

Fenugreek has a mild, somewhat nutty, not unpleasant taste. I have found the powder a good vehicle for mixing other herbs, vitamins, and minerals, especially for my pediatric diabetic patients. I recommend mixing the desired dosages of these other supplements into the fenugreek powder, and then mix it into a smoothie or other palatable food. Defatted fenugreek seed powder is available in some pharmacies and health food stores.

Table 2. Typical Dosage for Herbs

Herb	Typical Dosage
Gymnema sylvestre	400 to 600 mg standardized extract daily
Momordica charantia	100 to 200 mg standardized extract (0.5% charantin) 3 times daily
Trigonella foenum graecum	25 to 50 g daily

Other Herbs That May Lower Blood Sugar

Researchers are investigating other herbs that may have blood sugar–lowering properties. Elsewhere in the world, some of these herbs have been used for hundreds and even thousands of years as medicines or foods. I'll mention a few words about each. In many cases, the proper dose is not known precisely, so no recommendation is given.

Coccinia indica

In a double-blind, 6-week study of 32 diabetic patients, 16 received an herbal preparation from the leaves of *Coccinia indica,* an herb native to India and Bengal, used since ancient times by Ayurvedic physicians. Another group of 16 received a placebo. Ten of the 16 in the experimental group and none in the placebo group experienced marked improvement in blood sugar control.[21] Animal studies suggest that this herb lowers blood sugar in a manner similar to that of Momordica.[22]

Pterocarpus marsupium

Pterocarpus marsupium has a long history of medicinal use in India for a variety of maladies.

An open trial in four centers in India found this herb in doses from 2 to 4 g daily to be effective in lowering blood sugar in people with mild type 2 diabetes.[23] By 12 weeks, good blood sugar control had been attained in 67 (69%) of the 97 patients in the study. The necessary dose for maintaining good blood sugar control was 2 g in 73%, 3 g in 16%, and 4 g in 10% of patients.

Animal and test tube studies have also confirmed the blood sugar–lowering effect of this herb.[24, 25] Some preliminary studies found that extracts of epicatechin, a constituent of this plant, prevented beta cell destruction in animals given substances that can cause diabetes—and even regenerated destroyed pancreatic beta cells.[26] However, other studies have not found this isolated extract effective, even when it was injected directly into the pancreatic area[27, 28]

Perhaps using the entire Pterocarpus plant will prove more effective than using isolated extracts, but more research needs to be performed.

Formal safety studies of Pterocarpus have not been completed. For this reason, it cannot be recommended for young children, pregnant or nursing women, or people with severe liver or kidney disease.

Atriplex halimus (Salt Bush)

A study of plants used traditionally by people in Israel found 16 plants, including *Atriplex halimus* (salt bush), that had the potential to help control blood sugar levels in people with diabetes.[29] The body of information is growing concerning salt bush's effect on small mammals called sand rats, which get diabetes without it. However, the research on humans is limited to unpublished reports that blood glucose was lowered in type 2 diabetics who took salt bush daily.[30, 31]

Because no formal safety studies of salt bush have been conducted, the herb cannot be recommended for young children, pregnant or nursing women, or people with severe liver or kidney disease.

Vaccinium myrtillus (Bilberry)

Bilberry is widely used as a possible preventive treatment for complications of diabetes, as we will see in chapter 6. Not as well known, however, is the fact that this herb may possibly help lower blood sugar. In animal studies, bilberry was found to decrease blood sugar by 26% and triglycerides

by 39%.[32] Dosage of the standardized extract (standardized to contain 25% anthocyanosides) is 80 to 160 mg, 3 times daily.

In animal studies, bilberry was found to decrease blood sugar by 26% and triglycerides by 39%.

Bilberry is a widely eaten food that is closely related to the American blueberry. As a food it is quite safe. Since the concentrated extracts may have different properties than the whole fruit, I will remind you that the herb's safety has not been established for young children, pregnant or nursing women, or people with severe liver or kidney disease. However, there are no known or suspected problems with such uses.

Syzygium cucumi

Syzygium cucumi (jambol) is often touted as an effective herb for lowering blood sugar. However, a search of the literature uncovered one study performed on diabetic rats in which jambol was ineffective, administered in dosages equivalent to those sometimes used in humans.[33] The only studies on blood sugar effects in humans were not done on people with diabetes.

Foods That May Help Lower Blood Sugar

Did you know that certain foods contain chemicals that might help lower blood sugar? Researchers are beginning to study these foods, which include onions, garlic, and Jerusalem artichokes. However, most of the research is extremely preliminary.

Onions

Onions and garlic are two relatives with similar properties. Onions contain a substance called allyl propyl disulphide (APDS), and garlic contains diallyl disulfide oxide (allicin). These two substances may lower blood sugar by inhibiting the inactivation of insulin in the liver.[34]

A search of the literature revealed a few studies on the effect of onion extracts on blood sugar. However, only one was actually conducted on human diabetics, and it included only three subjects.[35] In this study, an onion extract was found to decrease the rise of blood sugar that occurs after a meal.

Inulin

Jerusalem artichokes, burdock root, and dandelion contain a substance called inulin, which can help lower blood sugar after a meal. Inulin from Jerusalem artichoke was found to slow the usual rise in blood sugar after a meal in normal, nondiabetic subjects,[36] probably by slowing absorption of glucose in the intestine. Powdered burdock root, given to diabetics in the form of crackers, inhibited the expected blood sugar rise after a starchy meal.[37]

Clinical Observations

I'd like to supplement the scientific evidence in this chapter with a few more experiences from my clinical practice. While this personal clinical experience isn't as reliable as scientific study results, it may be useful for people who wish to try these herbs.

Audrey's Story: Improved Blood Sugar Control

Audrey came to see me during the first year of my practice as a naturopathic physician. She was having trouble losing weight, as well as experiencing other health problems. I was able to help her with some chronic digestive and skin problems, but was not particularly successful helping her with the weight. She eventually went on one of those liquid protein, no-fat diets, lost about 100 pounds, and gained a gallbladder full of stones. Over the years her weight see-sawed, and she eventually gained back all the weight she had lost and more.

One day she came to see me, and told me she had recently been diagnosed with type 2 diabetes. Rather than prescribe medication, her medical doctor suggested she control her diet and lose some weight. I recommended some dietary changes as well, and put her on an herbal formula containing Gymnema, Momordica, and fenugreek to help lower her blood sugar.

Audrey tested her blood sugar at home, but not on a regular basis. Because of this, I decided the best way to determine how well she was in control was to test her glycosylated hemoglobin (HbA1c) at the beginning of treatment and about 3 months later. Before she began to take the herbal formula, her HbA1c was high—8.2. At the end of 3 months, however, it was 5.3—normal. She did not make dramatic changes in her diet, but she did cut back on desserts. Although it's impossible to be certain what contribution the herbal formula made to the improved blood sugar control, the overall effect was highly satisfactory. In thinking about that formula, I believe the Gymnema and Momordica had the most dramatic effect, as the fenugreek in the formula was in a smaller dose than is typically used for blood sugar lowering.

Conflicting Results with the Same Herb

Several years ago, a friend and colleague of mine returned from India with some *Coccinia indica*, an herb described above. Researchers he knew had done some preliminary studies on animals, and found that the herb appeared to regenerate beta cells in the pancreas. My colleague, who had type 1 diabetes, decided to try the herb himself. He took the recommended dosage—15 drops of the liquid tincture 4 times daily, before each meal and at bedtime. To his delight, he found he was able to decrease his insulin dosage by about one-third after a few weeks of taking the herb.

I shared this information with Joe, one of my patients who was having significant problems controlling his blood sugar. Joe was quite interested in trying it. At the time, *Coccinia indica* was not available in this country, so I ordered some from the doctor in India who was doing the research. Surprisingly, it seemed to *increase* Joe's insulin requirement! We soon discontinued it. Joe and I have tried other herbs over the years, including Gymnema, Momordica, and Syzygium. In each case, the herb seemed to increase his insulin requirement.

My thought—and it is just a hypothesis—is that the herbs may somehow be competing with the insulin he is injecting, taking up valuable insulin binding sites on the cells. There is still much we don't know about how these natural treatments really work

QUICK REVIEW

- Herbal approaches may have something to offer in treating diabetes, but the scientific research is sketchy and not well documented. Most of it has been conducted in India, where herbs have been used this way for thousands of years.

- The most well-studied herbs are *Gymnema sylvestre* (400 to 600 mg standardized extract daily), *Momordica charantia,* also known as bitter melon, (2 ounces fresh juice or 300 to 600 mg standardized extract), and fenugreek (25 to 50 g daily).

- Other herbs, used traditionally but with fewer supportive studies, are *Coccinia indica, Pterocarpus marsupium,* salt bush, and *Syzygium cucumi.* Bilberry has several studies supporting its effect relative to complications of diabetes (see chapter 6), but we have only animal studies to suggest that it might lower blood sugar too.

- A number of common foods also demonstrate some blood sugar–lowering possibilities, although the evidence is still very weak. These include onion, garlic, and Jerusalem artichoke.

- None of these treatments is sufficiently powerful to replace insulin for type 1 diabetics. However, they may be able to lower insulin needs and perhaps replace oral medications in type 2 diabetes.

- Always have medical supervision when you use these herbs to avoid lowering blood sugar levels too far and get help in adjusting medication dosages as necessary.

- Most of the herbs mentioned in this chapter have not been subjected to comprehensive formal safety studies. In particular, safety has not been established in young children, pregnant or nursing women, or people with severe liver or kidney disease.

Preventing Diabetic Nerve Damage

I n the past, many people with diabetes died from the immediate consequences of uncontrolled blood sugar. However, since the development of insulin, it is the long-term complications that have become the greatest problem for people with diabetes. One of the most debilitating of these complications is diabetic neuropathy, a syndrome of progressive nerve damage.

Several natural supplements may be useful for this condition. While none are solidly proven, some good evidence supports at least two treatments for diabetic nerve damage that are widely used in Europe: lipoic acid and essential fatty acids. There are several other supplements that may help as well.

Note: As you read this chapter, keep in mind that the most important step you can take is to control your blood sugar as well as possible.

Dwayne's Story

When the doctor diagnosed him with type 2 diabetes 5 years ago, it came as a total surprise to Dwayne. He hadn't been aware of anything unusual. Sure, he got up a couple of times a night to go to the bathroom, but didn't most middle-aged men? At first it was hard for him to take his diabetes seriously. He didn't try very hard to lose weight or follow his diet. His doctor lectured him about complications, but he didn't really believe they would happen to him.

Last year, though, Dwayne began to notice something unusual. His feet were becoming numb. Sometimes he felt as if he were wearing shoes when he was barefoot. He just didn't seem to have the sensation he was used to having. The doctor told Dwayne he was experiencing the beginnings of nerve damage from his diabetes and warned him not to go barefoot and to examine his feet nightly for injuries he might not have

What Is Diabetic Neuropathy?

If you are diabetic, chances are you've already heard of diabetic neuropathy, the damage to nerves that can develop in both types of diabetes. As you may know, it most commonly causes numbness, tingling, and pain in the legs, feet, and sometimes the arms and hands. Neuropathy can cause muscle weakness in these areas as well. The pain can sometimes be severe; when pain is severe, it often disappears after months or years and is replaced by numbness. The nerves responsible for these symptoms occur in the extremities or "periphery" of the body, rather than in the brain and spinal cord, so these symptoms are said to be due to *diabetic peripheral neuropathy.*

There's another kind of diabetic neuropathy you may not have heard of, called *diabetic autonomic neuropathy.*

been aware of. Dwayne's physician told him the risk of infection was great from unnoticed cuts or sores.

These symptoms of nerve damage were a wake-up call to Dwayne. For the first time, he began to seriously watch his diet and monitor his blood sugar, to help prevent the worsening of his condition. He also wanted to know whether he could do something to decrease the symptoms he was having.

Dwayne's doctor mentioned that a medical colleague in Germany was prescribing lipoic acid for symptoms such as these. Dwayne did some research and decided to try lipoic acid. He's now on a regime of lipoic acid, vitamins, minerals, and essential fatty acids. It's too early to tell, but Dwayne hopes these will help bring back sensation in his feet. This chapter will reveal the scientific evidence that can tell us whether Dwayne is right.

It affects nerves to body parts that are not normally under conscious control: the heart, intestines, blood vessels, and so on. Symptoms depend on what internal organ is affected. If the nerves to the intestines are involved, the result may be constipation, diarrhea, or both in succession. If the heart nerves are affected, the person may experience disturbances in the heart rate and rhythm. Autonomic neuropathy can also cause impotence, low blood pressure when standing up (called postural hypotension), and inability to sweat.

What Causes Diabetic Neuropathy?

Theories abound as to what causes diabetic complications, including neuropathy. Consistently elevated blood sugar levels seem to be the principal problem, but most likely, more than one factor is responsible. I will discuss several prominent theories here, along with the natural preventive treatments that may relate to them.

Sorbitol—Danger Within the Cell

Sorbitol is a by-product of glucose or galactose (another sugar), and may be associated with diabetic neuropathy. It is produced when glucose or galactose come in contact with an enzyme called *aldose reductase*. High blood sugar can lead to an overabundance of sorbitol, which in turn can build up within nerve cells and damage them. I'll explain in a little more detail how this can happen.

Ordinarily, insulin controls the entry of sugar into cells. However, glucose and galactose can enter nerve cells (as well as some other cells) even without insulin. Once they are inside, aldose reductase converts them to sorbitol, which can't leak back out because of the way it is made. As sorbitol accumulates inside the cells, chemical forces cause water to flow into the cells as well. The extra water makes the cells swell. Some scientists believe this swelling of nerve cells is one cause of neuropathy.[1]

The most important method to prevent this damage is to lower blood sugar levels. If the blood contains less glucose, less will travel into cells to be turned into sorbitol. Also, since it's aldose reductase that converts glucose and galactose to sorbitol, an obvious possible approach is to block the action of aldose reductase. Substances that can do this are called *aldose reductase inhibitors.* Animal studies have found various aldose reductase inhibitor drugs to improve nerve conduction in diabetic neuropathy.[2] However, most of them seem to cause too many side effects.

Vitamin C also appears to inhibit aldose reductase, and some practitioners suggest it as a side-effect-free alternative to these drugs. However, since vitamin C is more often suggested as a treatment for diabetic eye disease, you'll find it discussed in the next chapter. Alpha lipoic acid, a treatment for diabetic neuropathy widely used in Europe, may also function by inhibiting aldose reductase. This will be discussed in more detail later in the chapter.

Fighting Free Radicals

Some of the chief suspects in diabetic neuropathy are known as "free radicals." These substances can damage many tissues, including the lipids (fats) in nerve cells. Damage to fats caused by free radicals is called lipid peroxidation. In test tube studies, researchers found lipid peroxidation to be increased in experimental diabetic neuropathy.[3] Supplements that can help neutralize free radicals are called antioxidants. They include lipoic acid, vitamin E, and selenium, among others.

Some of the chief suspects in diabetic neuropathy are known as "free radicals."

Other Theories Behind Diabetic Neuropathy

Sorbitol buildup also results in a decrease in inositol,[4] a nutrient important for proper nerve function that's loosely associated with the B-complex family of vitamins. Low inositol interferes with an enzyme necessary for proper nerve conduction, and several animal studies suggest this may be a factor in diabetic neuropathy.[5, 6]

Finally, evidence points to decreased blood flow to the nerves in diabetic neuropathy.[7] This too may contribute to the development of nerve damage in diabetes. Some natural supplements may help increase blood flow as well.

Natural Prevention and Treatment of Diabetic Neuropathy

One good thing about diabetic neuropathy—if anything good can be said about it—is that it takes years to develop. Unfortunately, this poses a problem for studying natural prevention of this condition. Only a few human studies have been completed on natural approaches to diabetic neuropathy, most of which were fairly short term. Some longer-term studies presently under way should give us more information about effective natural remedies.

Alpha Lipoic Acid—Widely Used in Germany

Alpha lipoic acid, sometimes called thioctic acid, is a vital substance produced in the body. Diabetes may reduce levels of lipoic acid in the body.[8] However, this in itself does not mean that taking lipoic acid supplements will reduce symptoms. You need direct studies to show that lipoic acid supplements will increase levels in the body. Fortunately, researchers have conducted several studies, and the results have been strong enough to make lipoic acid a widely used treatment in Germany for the past two decades.

In practice, lipoic acid appears to be fairly effective. As one patient said, "After I took lipoic acid for a couple of weeks, I could feel my feet again. It wasn't completely back to normal, but it was a big improvement." Other patients report that lipoic acid can "take the edge off" when diabetic neuropathy causes pain instead of numbness.

What Is the Scientific Evidence for Lipoic Acid?

Studies show promise for lipoic acid in reducing both pain and numbness due to diabetic neuropathy. One of the largest studies on lipoic acid looked at 328 type 2 diabetics with symptoms of neuropathy, including pain.[9] In this double-blind study, subjects received either 1,200, 600, or 100 mg lipoic acid or placebo intravenously every day. Subjects completed pain score questionnaires at the study's beginning and end. The 1,200 and 600 mg groups had significantly less pain than did the people taking the placebo. Those taking 600 mg experienced the most improvement.

While this study is promising, we must note that it lasted only 3 weeks and participants received the lipoic acid intravenously, not by mouth. However, lipoic acid is well-absorbed orally, and other studies showed oral doses were effective.

Another controlled (but not blinded) study looked at decreased sensation rather than pain.[10] Eighty type 1 or type 2 diabetics with neuropathy were divided into four groups: One group received 600 mg of oral lipoic acid daily, one group received placebo, and two groups received other antioxidants: either 1,200 IU vitamin E or 100 mcg of selenium daily. Researchers measured changes in participants' sensitivity to temperature and vibration. After 3

Studies show promise for lipoic acid in reducing both pain and numbness due to diabetic neuropathy.

months, all the groups receiving the antioxidants showed significant improvement in sensation compared to the placebo group. Of particular note, this study suggests the possibility of equally significant benefits using more common, cheaper antioxidants.

Lipoic acid also may be helpful for autonomic neuropathy. As I noted above, this condition affects nerves to organs controlling the "unconscious" processes of the body—heart rate, digestion, and so on. A 4-month, double-blind, placebo-controlled study tested lipoic acid in treating cardiac autonomic neuropathy (CAN) of diabetes.[11] This condition is caused by damage to nerves controlling the heart, causing people to faint when they stand up, among other symptoms. In the study, 29 diabetics with CAN received oral doses of 800 mg lipoic acid daily, while 27 took a placebo. The people taking lipoic acid had significant improvement in irregular heart rate compared to those in the placebo group.

How Does Lipoic Acid Work?

Lipoic acid may work in more ways than one, but the most important way is probably as an antioxidant. Test-tube studies have found lipoic acid to decrease free radical damage in nerve cells.[12] As I mentioned earlier, free radical damage may be one way diabetes injures nerves. The study I mentioned above[13] showed that three different antioxidants, including lipoic acid, were all effective in improving symptoms of neuropathy.

Studies have also shown lipoic acid to inhibit aldose reductase.[14] You may remember that aldose reductase inhibitors may protect nerve cells by helping prevent dangerous accumulation of sorbitol.

Animal studies have also shown a 50% decrease in blood flow to the nerves after diabetes develops. Intravenous administration of lipoic acid reversed these changes, restoring the speed of nerve conduction to normal after 3 months of treatment.[15] So it's possible that lipoic acid may also work in part by improving blood flow to nerves.

Dosage

The therapeutic oral dose of lipoic acid appears to be in the range of 600 to 800 mg daily.

Warning: Do not inject lipoic acid meant for oral use.

Safety Issues

Formal safety studies of lipoic acid have not been completed. Nonetheless, during 3 decades of study and clinical use in Germany, no serious adverse effects have been reported. Because comprehensive data is lacking, however, lipoic acid use is not advised during pregnancy.[16] Safety in young children and people with severe liver or kidney disease has also not been established.

High doses of lipoic acid (20 mg/kg) have been found to be toxic to rats deficient in thiamin (vitamin B_1).[17] Supplementing with thiamin reversed this effect. While the effect has not been noted in human studies, you may be well advised to take 50 mg or so of B_1 (or a B complex containing B_1) when using lipoic acid.

Allergic reactions to lipoic acid occur occasionally. There have also been reports of hypoglycemia due to improved glucose utilization.[18] For this and other reasons, diabetics should seek medical supervision before taking lipoic acid.

Essential Fatty Acids—
A Source of Gamma-Linolenic Acid

Perhaps the most common dietary advice you hear these days is to eat less fat. Researchers have discovered that fat increases the incidence of a great many diseases, including the big three killers: cancer, heart disease, and strokes.

However, not all fat is bad. Saturated fats, found in milk, beef, animal products and certain vegetable oils certainly do seem to be harmful. However, some unsaturated fats seem to be good for you. Certain fats, called essential fatty acids (EFAs) appear to be as essential as vitamins. Just like vitamin C deficiency causes scurvy, severe deficiencies of EFAs can lead to dry skin, hair loss, eczema, decreased immunity, and arthritis. Evidence suggests that supplemental doses of an EFA called gamma-linolenic acid (GLA) may be able to reduce the symptoms of diabetic neuropathy.

Ordinarily, your body can make GLA from linoleic acid, a more common essential fatty acid found in most vegetable oils. Research suggests, however, that people with diabetes may have trouble converting linoleic acid to GLA. For this reason, GLA supplements may be a good idea. Natural sources of GLA include evening primrose oil, black currant oil, and borage oil. Although evening primrose oil has been studied the most extensively, black currant and borage oils have higher percentages of important GLA.

While GLA seems to act more slowly than lipoic acid, some good evidence suggests that it may be effective if used long enough. Animal studies suggest that the combination may be more effective still, but this has not been proven in humans.

What Is the Scientific Evidence for GLA?

Research on GLA generally shows it to be effective in diabetic neuropathy when taken for a long period—3 to 6 months. I'll discuss two of the more recent studies here.

One double-blind, placebo-controlled study involved 111 patients with mild diabetic neuropathy. Patients received either 480 mg GLA or placebo daily for 1 year.[19] Researchers used 16 measurements to evaluate their neuropathy: sensation, tendon reflexes, muscle strength, and so on. The GLA group did significantly better than the placebo group in 13 of these measurements.

A smaller double-blind study of 22 diabetics with neuropathy compared the effects of a placebo to 4 g daily evening primrose oil (EPO), which is the equivalent of 360 mg GLA.[20] After 6 months, all eight variables that were monitored had improved in the evening primrose oil group but worsened in the placebo group.

In general, we still have a lot to learn about how supplements interact with each other. However, in this case, animal studies suggest that GLA and lipoic acid work well together.[21, 22] GLA appears to work partly by increasing blood flow to the nerves.[23, 24]

Dosage

In the few human studies, dosage ranged from 360 to 480 mg GLA daily—about 4 to 5 g of evening primrose oil, which is 9% GLA. If you're using borage or black currant oil, you may be able to use less since they contain 24% and 18% GLA respectively.

As with all oil products, once you open the bottle, be sure to store it in a cool, dark place (such as the refrigerator) to avoid rancidity. Products in gel caps are less likely to become rancid than the free-flowing oil.

Safety Issues

Most of the safety studies that apply to GLA have been performed using evening primrose oil. In animal studies, evening primrose oil appears to be nontoxic and noncarcinogenic,[25] and does not seem to cause birth defects.

Because GLA has been widely studied for a number of conditions, we have more safety information for this essential fatty acid than for some other natural remedies. More than 4,000 patients have participated in studies of GLA, mostly in the form of EPO. No adverse effects have been attributed to this treatment, and double-blind studies of EPO have shown no significant differences in rate of side effects between the treated group and the placebo group.[26] In addition, the U.K. National Health Service had issued more than 500,000 prescriptions of EPO by 1992, with no definite reports of adverse effects linked to EPO. However, somewhat fewer than 2% of patients who take evening primrose oil complain of headaches, mild gastrointestinal distress, or both—especially at higher doses.[27, 28]

While lipoic acid and evening primrose oil have a significant level of evidence behind them, the treatments described in the rest of this chapter are fairly speculative.

Acetyl L-Carnitine

Acetyl L-carnitine, a form of the amino acid L-carnitine, is synthesized in the body. It appears to protect nerves in both the central nervous system (brain and spinal cord) and the extremities.

What Is the Scientific Evidence for Acetyl L-Carnitine?

The human studies of acetyl L-carnitine used an injected form of the supplement. Properly designed human studies using oral forms of the supplement have not yet been completed, and until they are we cannot say whether the oral form is effective or not.

A small double-blind study found acetyl L-carnitine injections effective for the pain of diabetic neuropathy.[29] In another double-blind trial on patients with neuropathy (not necessarily all from diabetes), 31 received 500 mg daily of acetyl L-carnitine by injection, 32 received 1,000 mg daily acetyl-L-carnitine also by injection, and 31 received placebo.[30] After 15 days, patients on acetyl L-carnitine had less pain and better nerve function than did those taking placebo.

Animal studies have also pointed to some potential effectiveness of acetyl L-carnitine. It was found to speed up nerve conduction to normal levels in diabetic rats.[31]

How Does Acetyl L-Carnitine Work?

Studies on this supplement are still in the early stages. Some researchers have found it to increase lowered inositol levels as well as reduce free radical damage.[32] As I mentioned above, decreased inositol may be a contributing factor in diabetic neuropathy, and free radical damage is another suspected cause.

Dosage

It may be too early to determine the optimum dosage for oral administration of this supplement. When given intramuscularly, the optimum dosage appeared to be approximately 1,000 mg (1 g) daily.

Warning: Do not inject acetyl L-carnitine designed for oral use—it is not safe.

The optimum oral dosage of this supplement for diabetic neuropathy is not known. When it is used for other therapeutic purposes such as Alzheimer's disease, typical doses are in the range of 1.5 to 3 g daily. (For more information on acetyl L-carnitine as a treatment for Alzheimer's disease, see *The Natural Pharmacist Guide to Ginkgo and Memory*.)

Safety Issues

No serious side effects have been reported in humans, but researchers have not yet completed formal safety testing. Most study of acetyl L-carnitine has involved nondiabetics. Studies have shown the supplement to decrease the metabolism of alcohol in animals, keeping it in the body longer, but at the same time decreasing damage to the liver.

In studies for Alzheimer's disease after 3 months, 11% of patients reported increased agitation (which decreased to 7% after 6 months), compared to 6% in a placebo group.[33] Nausea has also been reported occasionally.

Safety in young children, pregnant or nursing women, or people with severe liver or kidney disease has not been established.

B Complex Family of Vitamins— Promising but No Hard Facts

Researchers have looked at several members of the B-complex family of vitamins to see whether they could help with diabetic neuropathy. These include B_1 (thiamin), B_6 (pyridoxine), B_{12} (cobalamin), inositol, and pantethine (the active form of B_5). So far only preliminary evidence suggests that any of these help, and some evidence suggests they might not help. I'll briefly review information on each in turn.

Vitamin B_1 (Thiamin)

Stanley Mirsky, MD, past president of the New York branch of the American Diabetes Association, observed that about 80% of his diabetic patients with neuropathy were helped with thiamin supplements. However, little scientific evidence supports this suggestion. I'm aware of only one double-blind, controlled study of B_1 in diabetic neuropathy, and that study combined thiamin with B_6 and B_{12}. In this study of 24 patients, the vitamin group showed a significant improvement in the speed of nerve conduction after 12 weeks when compared to the placebo group.[34]

Vitamin B_6 (Pyridoxine)

B_6 deficiency can cause symptoms of neuropathy even without diabetes. Since some researchers have found diabetics, particularly those with neuropathy, to be deficient in B_6,[35] some practitioners suggest that certain cases of apparent diabetic neuropathy are actually B_6 deficiency in disguise. But so far no high-quality studies have backed this up. In fact, one study of 119 diabetics (53 with neuropathy and 66 without) found no important differences in vitamin status between those who had neuropathy and those who didn't.[36]

Furthermore, in a double-blind study with 18 subjects, improvement in symptoms of neuropathy was no better in the group taking 50 mg of B_6 3 times daily than in those taking the placebo.[37]

Vitamin B_{12} (Cobalamin)

Levels of vitamin B_{12} may be low in patients with diabetic neuropathy,[38] although not all studies agree.[39] Several small clinical observations with 5 to 12 patients have shown benefit.[40–42] In these studies, patients received intramuscular injections of B_{12} ranging from 2,500

Some practitioners suggest that certain cases of apparent diabetic neuropathy are actually B_6 deficiency in disguise.

mcg several days in a row to low doses of 15 to 30 mcg daily. However, because these trials were not double-blinded and lacked a control group, the results aren't reliable.

Inositol

Some scientists have postulated that decreased inositol may have a role in diabetic neuropathy, perhaps by slowing down nerve conduction. Remember our discussion of acetyl L-carnitine? One theory is that acetyl L-carnitine works by increasing inositol. So it makes sense that scientists would consider supplementing inositol directly. In one small, unblinded study, patients with neuropathy received 500 mg inositol twice daily for 2 weeks.[43] Some signs of neuropathy improved significantly, while others did not.

Other studies have not been so promising. Twenty-eight diabetics who were just beginning to show signs of neuropathy took 6 g daily of inositol or placebo for 2 months. What was the result? No difference in signs of

Rachel's Story

I have been seeing Rachel, a diabetes patient, for about 8 years. She is 45 years old and was diagnosed with type 1 diabetes in her early 20s. Her primary complication is neuropathy, which has mainly consisted of numbness in her feet and shooting leg pains, especially at night. Over the years, as I learn of new possible therapies, I suggest them to Rachel. She is taking a lot of supplements, including lipoic acid (300 mg twice daily), pantethine (200 mg twice daily), B-complex (50 mg twice daily), EFAs (combination of borage and fish oil—3 g daily), and acetyl L-carnitine (1,000 mg twice daily). Because the supplements have been added slowly over the years, and the symptoms of the neuropathy have also changed slowly, determining whether the supplements were making a big difference or not, or which ones were the most effective, has been difficult.

Recently Rachel called and told me this story. She had gone for a short trip into New York City from her home in Connecticut. She had planned to stay just a day or two so had taken only her multiple vitamin. While in New York she was offered some possible job opportunities and ended up staying two weeks for interviews—and to shop. After about a week to ten days without the remainder of her supple-

neurological function between the two groups was observed.[44]

Vitamin B$_5$ (Pantethine)

Pantethine is the active form of vitamin B$_5$ or pantothenic acid. Sixteen patients with diabetic neuropathy were

ments, she began having shooting leg pains—something she had forgotten about. She wondered whether it was due to the lack of her usual supplements. When she got back to Connecticut, she resumed her usual supplement regime and her leg pains subsided. Her numbness, on the other hand, has persisted throughout the treatment, whether she's on supplements or not.

Prior to this event, Rachel and I had wondered whether the supplements were actually helping the pain or whether the neuropathy had simply progressed past the pain stage to total numbness. In her case, they appear to help the pain. Keep in mind that although Rachel did well with them, we don't know for sure whether combining separate treatments for diabetic neuropathy produces better results than using one treatment or another. As I mentioned above, some evidence supports combining lipoic acid and GLA, and it certainly stands to reason that the other treatment might work in combination, also. When you start mixing numerous treatments together, however, you run the risk that one treatment may counteract another. Rachel and I look forward to the day when much more is known about these remedies, individually and as a group.

given varying dosages of pantethine, ranging from 30 to 200 mg daily.[45] Pantethine supplementation improved pain in 33% of cases and reflexes in 40% of cases. However, double-blind, controlled studies still need to be conducted to determine whether pantethine actually works consistently.

It appears that the B vitamins, at least to the extent that they are correcting a possible deficiency, may have some application in the treatment of diabetic neuropathy, although scientifically meaningful clinical trials have yet to be conducted. However, because the B vitamins are readily available and nontoxic for the most part, there is no reason for you to avoid supplementation. Do note, though, that B_6 in large doses—150 mg daily and above—has sometimes been found to actually cause symptoms of neuropathy.

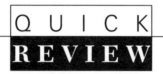

QUICK
REVIEW

- Nerve damage, or diabetic neuropathy, is a frequent long-term complication of diabetes.

- The two basic types are peripheral neuropathy (which you may notice as pain, numbness, and tingling in arms, hands, legs, or feet) and autonomic neuropathy (which affects nerves supplying organs and can disrupt digestion, heart rate, or other unconscious bodily processes).

- We don't know all the causes of neuropathy. It may be partly a result of sorbitol accumulation in the nerve cells, which results in a decline in the inositol levels. Free radical damage has also been implicated.

- A number of natural substances have been found by some investigators to be effective in preventing and treating diabetic neuropathy.

    Among the most well-researched are lipoic acid, a natural antioxidant, (300 mg twice daily) and gamma linolenic acid or GLA, an essential fatty acid. A dosage for GLA is 250 mg twice daily—about 5 g of evening primrose oil, which is 9% GLA. If you're using borage or black currant oil, you may be able to use less since they contain 24% and 18% GLA, respectively.

Other substances that hold promise for the treatment of neuropathy include acetyl L-carnitine (An optimum oral dosage is approximately 1,000 mg twice daily. See chapter for safety warnings.) and the active form of B_5 pantethine (see dosage below).

- Some diabetics with neuropathy may be deficient in certain B vitamins such as B_1, B_6, B_{12}, and inositol. Correcting the deficiency may improve symptoms of neuropathy. Taking a good B complex vitamin providing about 100 mg B_1 and B_6, and 1 mg of B_{12} daily should provide adequate amounts of the B vitamins. Inositol may be taken at a dosage of 500 mg twice daily, and pantethine 200 mg twice daily.

Diabetic Eye Complications

A s we have seen throughout this book, consistently elevated blood sugar levels cause damage to many parts of the body. This chapter discusses the various diabetes-related eye conditions. The most devastating vision problem is retinopathy. Cataracts, too, are more common among people with diabetes than among the population at large. Fortunately, as you will see, you can take some natural steps to help keep your eyes healthy, even if you have diabetes. But don't forget that good blood sugar control is the most important step you can take.

What Is Retinopathy?

Retinopathy is the term for damage to the retina—the area at the back of the eye that records images and converts them into signals to be sent to the brain. Retinopathy is a devastating complication of diabetes that can lead to blindness. The risk of diabetic retinopathy is directly related to the number of years a person has had diabetes, and how well or poorly the blood sugar has been controlled. Promising research indicates that supplements, including vitamins, bilberry, and lipoic acid, may also help slow or prevent this debilitating condition. Diabetic retinopathy begins with damage to the blood vessels in the eye. Leakage from capillaries is one of the first signs, followed by swelling, blockage of vessels, and small hemorrhages. This stage is called "background retinopathy." If swelling occurs in the region of the macula, the most sensitive part of the retina, the resulting loss of vision may be serious and possibly permanent.

Retinopathy is a devastating complication of diabetes that can lead to blindness.

In about 10 to 20% of cases, background retinopathy goes on to become "proliferative retinopathy." In this condition, the retina tries to compensate for lack of oxygen by forming more blood vessels. Unfortunately, these fragile new vessels bleed easily, leading to scars that can distort the retina, sometimes pulling it from the back of the eye. Retinal detachment or hemorrhage can cause what is often the first symptom of retinopathy: sudden loss of vision in one eye.

Ophthalmologists commonly treat proliferative retinopathy with laser therapy. While highly effective, this treatment isn't a cure—the disease can still get worse. That's why using preventive strategies is so important.

What Causes Diabetic Retinopathy?

We don't completely understand the causes of retinopathy, but there are some solid theories. We'll explore some

Paul's Story

Paul was a proofreader. His vision was critical to his livelihood as well as to the one hobby that gave him most pleasure in life: photography. A type 1 diabetic since age 16, he was meticulous in his self-care. However, a series of hypoglycemic attacks persuaded Paul to keep his blood sugar a little above the normal range.

Paul followed all his endocrinologist's guidelines for protecting his vision. He didn't smoke, kept his blood pressure normal, and had his eyes checked for signs of retinopathy every year by an ophthalmologist. However, the day came when the eye doctor told Paul he was beginning to develop

of them here and show how they relate to natural treatments a bit later in the chapter.

Glycosylated Proteins and Free Radicals

One cause of many diabetic complications, including retinopathy, is the formation of *glycosylated proteins* and the resulting production of free radicals.[1] Remember our discussion in chapter 3 of glycosylated hemoglobin used to test long-term blood sugar control? Over time, if blood sugar is high, glucose can attach to proteins such as hemoglobin. When this happens, we say the protein is "glycosylated." Hemoglobin is just one of the proteins that can become glycosylated.

Glycosylated proteins can generate *free radicals,* which cause what is called "oxidative stress," resulting in tissue damage. The body manufactures substances called antioxidants to neutralize free radicals. In the presence of too many free radicals, these natural neutralizers can become depleted.

damage to the retina of his eye. The damage was not enough to cause symptoms or require treatment, but was enough to make Paul worry. Paul knew that he was now at higher risk for a more severe stage of retinopathy—one that could lead to a sudden loss of vision if not attended to promptly.

So Paul began pursuing alternatives he hoped would prevent more retinal damage. He researched natural treatments such as vitamin C and bilberry, and began a program under the supervision of his ophthalmologist. The eye doctor supported him in taking any safe steps that might help protect his vision.

Here's some of the evidence that free radicals may contribute to retinopathy. One of these natural antioxidants, an enzyme called *glutathione,* has been found to be deficient in the retinas of diabetic rats and dogs.[2] This suggests that depleted defenses against free radicals can play a part in the development of retinopathy. To further support this theory, diabetics with retinopathy appear to have more of a certain chemical (malondialdehyde) that increases during oxidative stress. In one study, diabetics with retinopathy had significantly more of this chemical than either diabetics without retinopathy or healthy control group participants.[3]

Besides contributing to oxidative stress, a subgroup of glycosylated proteins may cause further damage. Remember that glycosylated proteins are proteins gummed up with sugar? Some of them, called advanced glycated end-products (AGE) are themselves damaged by free radicals and also by combining with fats. They deposit in blood vessels and other tissues, wreaking all sorts of havoc. AGE appear to contribute to the growth of new blood vessels in proliferative retinopathy. Antioxidants may partially inhibit this process.[4] We'll look at the evidence for supplementing with natural antioxidant vitamins later in this chapter.

Lack of Oxygen to the Retina

In diabetic retinopathy, oxygen supply to parts of the retina is decreased. This is primarily caused by blocked blood vessels. Furthermore, the red blood cells of people with diabetes may be less flexible, particularly among those who have trouble keeping their blood sugar under control. The red blood cells need to change shape to fit through the tiny capillaries in the retina. If they can't do this, they may get stuck inside the narrowed vessels and create blockages, further reducing oxygen supply to certain areas of the retina. To compensate for the decreased oxygen, new blood vessels form, leading to the condition described above called proliferative retinopathy.

Sorbitol Accumulation

Researchers disagree as to whether accumulation of sorbitol, a glucose by-product, is a cause of retinopathy. Substances called aldose reductase inhibitors, which prevent accumulation of sorbitol, have been found to prevent retinopathy in studies of animals, but not in humans. See chapter 5 and the section on cataracts later in this chapter for more information on sorbitol.

Elevated Homocysteine Levels

Are elevated homocysteine levels associated with diabetic retinopathy? This is yet another area of controversy.

You may have heard about homocysteine in the news recently. If elevated in the bloodstream, this amino acid can contribute to heart problems. Some researchers think homocysteine may also contribute to retinopathy, although the evidence is conflicting.

In a study reported in the *Lancet*, homocysteine levels were tested in 25 patients with diabetes, 12 with retinopathy and 13 without.[5] The patients with retinopathy had abnormally high homocysteine levels, while those without retinopathy did not. It is believed that homocysteine can damage blood vessels, and this may be another mechanism leading to retinopathy.

However, another group of researchers examining a larger group—79 people with diabetes and 46 healthy controls—found no correlation between retinopathy and high homocysteine levels except in the patients who also had kidney damage (nephropathy).[6]

Controlling Blood Sugar Is Key in Preventing Retinopathy

If you want to prevent retinopathy, research tells us that controlling your blood sugar is key. The Diabetes Control and Complications Trial (DCCT) was a long-term study of thousands of people with diabetes who depend on insulin.[7] Its main purpose was to determine whether tighter blood sugar control might help prevent retinopathy. Researchers compared the effect of conventional insulin therapy (taking two injections a day) with intensive insulin therapy (maintaining tighter control over blood sugar by testing frequently throughout the day and injecting smaller amounts). In the first few months of the study, tighter control seemed to worsen retinopathy in more patients than did the conventional approach; however, in the long term, better blood sugar control resulted in a large reduction in long-term risk of developing retinopathy. This was the first study of its kind, and resulted in widespread recommendations for tight blood sugar control as the first line of prevention of diabetic complications.

A recent study in the prestigious British medical journal, the *Lancet,* found that intensive blood sugar control could reduce the risk of developing damage to the small blood vessels in the retina and kidney by 25%.[8] This study, The United Kingdom Prospective Diabetes Study, is the largest, longest-running study of people with type 2 diabetes. It enrolled 5,200 people and gathered data between 1977 and 1998. After examining the results, endocrinologist Alan Garber commented: "There is no limit to the benefit you can achieve when you lower blood sugars."

The goal in diabetes treatment is to mimic the natural action of insulin as closely as possible. Unfortunately, many people with type 1 diabetes and some with type 2 have difficulty maintaining very tight glucose control. Until science has found a way to abolish the ups and downs of blood sugar, inevitable with current treatment, it makes sense to consider other ways to prevent complications—in addition to good blood sugar control.

Other Natural Preventives of Retinopathy

What natural treatments can be used to augment the benefits of good blood sugar control? Unfortunately, few long-term human studies have focused on the use of natural substances for the prevention and treatment of diabetic retinopathy. This means that much of what we will discuss in the next pages is theoretical—based on what we think *should* work from our knowledge of retinopathy and the effects of various supplements.

Vitamin C

Vitamin C is an important water-soluble antioxidant. In addition, it plays a key role in producing and repairing connective tissue—the main building material of blood vessels, skin, ligaments, and muscles.

What Are the Potential Benefits of Vitamin C for Retinopathy?

There are several theories as to why extra vitamin C might help prevent and treat retinopathy. Remember that diabetes may diminish oxygen supply to the retina, through blood vessel damage and scarring. One theory holds that this lack of oxygen in the retina causes free radicals to develop. They in turn deplete the retina of antioxidant vitamin C. Logically, supplementing with vitamin C might help restore depleted levels and maintain antioxidant activity in the retina.

In fact, several researchers have found that vitamin C levels are lower in people with diabetes than in nondiabetics, and lowest in diabetics with retinopathy.[9, 10] This does not prove that taking more vitamin C will make a difference, but it certainly does suggest this.

Vitamin C has also been found to reduce glycosylation of proteins, both in a test tube and in healthy humans given an oral dose.[11, 12] As I described above, glycosylation of proteins is believed to be a cause of diabetic complications.

Vitamin C's importance in connective-tissue formation and repair makes it an important nutrient for maintaining healthy blood vessels.[13] A deficiency of vitamin C may make blood vessels more likely to leak.[14] Leaky blood vessels in the retina can result in hemorrhage and scar formation. Even if vitamin C isn't deficient in the whole body, it may be deficient in the eye, due to local conditions. Taking extra vitamin C may help.

A placebo-controlled study of 12 diabetics with and without retinopathy showed that 1,000 mg daily of vitamin C decreased capillary fragility.[15] But in this 3-month study, no significant retinal changes were apparent in either the group given vitamin C or in the controls. Three months may not have been long enough to see significant changes.

Putting it all together, there is good reason to believe that vitamin C supplements may prevent or reverse damage to the retina, but we don't yet know for sure.

Dosage

The standard recommended dose of vitamin C to prevent retinopathy is in the range of 2 to 4 g daily (about 2,000 to 4,000 mg). Because this dose is higher than normal dietary intake, you should take it only on the advice of a physician.

Safety Issues

Vitamin C is a water-soluble vitamin that does not accumulate in the tissues. It appears to be a very safe vitamin. The most common side effect of high doses of vitamin C is diarrhea. If this occurs, reduce the dosage.

Antioxidant research has made it more apparent that a balance of various antioxidants is important. High doses of vitamin C should be consumed with other antioxidants, such as vitamin E, because each vitamin keeps the other in a proper non-oxidized state.

Pregnant women should probably not consume more than about 500 mg of vitamin C daily, except on the advice of a physician.

The optimum dosages of vitamin C for children aren't known, but for many medications the standard approach is to reduce the dose proportionately by the child's weight. If you assume an average adult weighs 150 pounds, a 50-pound child, for example, would take one-third the adult dose.

Warning: Always consult your physician before you give children with diabetes high doses of any vitamin or mineral.

Vitamin C is primarily eliminated via the kidneys, so people with kidney disease should avoid taking large doses. Although there have been warnings that vitamin C can contribute to kidney stone formation, no evidence supports this theory.[16]

Vitamin E

Vitamin E is another antioxidant that may be useful for diabetic retinopathy. This fat-soluble vitamin has potent antioxidant effects on fat-soluble tissues like cell membranes; and it also has important blood-thinning effects.[17]

What Are the Potential Benefits of Vitamin E in Retinopathy?

Several researchers have found levels of vitamin E to be lower in people with diabetes than in nondiabetics, and especially low in diabetics with retinopathy.[18] This is a similar finding to that regarding vitamin C, and many of the functions of vitamin C with respect to retinopathy apply to vitamin E as well. For instance, like vitamin C, vitamin E has potent antioxidant effects. Also like vitamin C, vitamin E appears to prevent protein glycosylation.[19]

Glycosylated proteins do some of their damage by becoming oxidized easily and converting to toxic substances. Both vitamin E and lipoic acid can inhibit this damaging process.[20] Vitamin E therefore seems to inhibit both the production and oxidation of glycosylated proteins.

As mentioned earlier, glutathione (an important natural antioxidant in the body) appears to be deficient in the retinas of diabetic dogs and rats.[21] These same researchers found supplementation with vitamins E and C restored glutathione levels in the retina of diabetic rats.

Recently, researchers have discovered that (at least in diabetic animals) the activity of a certain enzyme pathway is increased in the retina in response to high blood sugar.[22]

A Case of Bilberry, Please

Although little direct evidence supports the use of bilberry, the plant is widely used in Europe based primarily on patient reports of benefit. Recently I spoke to a fellow naturopathic physician in the United States who told me about one of her patients with diabetic retinopathy. Martin was 70 years old and had type 2 diabetes. Although he ate well, kept his blood sugar under fair control, and walked an hour every day, eventually he developed retinopathy that interfered with his vision. He could no longer read his alarm clock when lying in bed, even when he wore his glasses.

Martin consulted his naturopathic physician—my friend—who suggested he try bilberry in hopes of preventing further

This enzyme pathway goes by the intimidating name of the diacylglycerol protein kinase C pathway, or the DAG-PKC pathway for short. This increased enzyme activity appears to interfere with normal circulation to the retina. Researchers have found that vitamin E can normalize the activity of the DAG-PKC pathway, leading to improved retinal blood flow.

Vitamin E also inhibits platelet stickiness.[23] Platelets are central to the development of blood clots. Since blood clots in retinal vessels play a key role in diabetic retinopathy, this is another way in which vitamin E may make a difference. However, we don't have any direct evidence that vitamin E actually prevents damaging blood clots in the retina.

Dosage

Therapeutic dosage of vitamin E for an adult is in the range of 400 to 800 IU daily.

progression of the disease. Martin gladly tried it, and just 6 weeks later he returned with surprising news—he was able to see the large numbers on his clock just a little. Over the months the blurriness became less severe until eventually he was again able to read the clock from his bed without his glasses.

At his next eye exam, the doctor told Martin his vision had significantly improved. Martin was thrilled, and went out and bought a whole case of bilberry!

Anecdotes of this type, however encouraging, do not really prove anything.

Safety Issues

Vitamin E appears to be quite safe, even when taken in very high doses. However, it does present a few potential risks. Some researchers have found vitamin E to elevate already high blood pressure in some people. Always monitor your blood pressure when you begin taking supplemental vitamin E—particularly since high blood pressure has been linked to retinopathy. Vitamin E also has the potential to thin the blood, so seek a physician's advice before combining it with other blood thinning medications such as Coumadin (warfarin), heparin, or aspirin. Vitamin E might also conceivably interact with other natural supplements that possess a mild blood thinning effect, such as garlic and ginkgo.

Vaccinium myrtillus (Bilberry)

Bilberry, or European blueberry, is a plant in the same family as the blueberries we eat. This plant has a long history of use in the treatment of diabetes and its complications. It contains important flavonoid compounds known as anthocyanosides, which appear to have a special affinity for the eye, particularly the retina.

What Are the Potential Benefits of Bilberry for Diabetic Retinopathy?

Most investigations of bilberry have focused on its flavonoid components, the anthocyanosides. These components are potent antioxidants and have two other important effects. They strengthen connective tissue, such as is found in the retina,[24] and they decrease the leakiness and fragility of the blood vessels.[25] Bilberry and herbs containing flavonoids with capillary-strengthening properties are also used to slow fluid leakage in other diseases, such as varicose veins.

Unfortunately no blinded, controlled studies of the effects of bilberry on diabetic retinopathy have been conducted. A highly preliminary, unblinded human trial has been conducted with inconclusive results.[26] The researcher reported a trend toward decreased hemorrhage in retinopathy.

Dosage
Studies have generally been conducted with a standardized extract containing 25% anthocyanosides. The usual dosage of this extract is 80 to 160 mg 3 times daily.

Safety Issues
As one might expect of a food, bilberry is quite safe. Enormous quantities have been administered to rats without toxic effects.[27, 28] One study of 2,295 patients showed no serious side effects and only a 4% incidence of mild reactions such as gastrointestinal distress, skin rashes, and drowsiness.[29]

Safety in young children, pregnant or lactating women, or people with severe liver or kidney disease has not been established, although no known or suspected problems have been reported with such uses. It is possible, however, that the concentrated extracts may have different properties than the whole fruit.

L-Carnitine

As you learned in chapter 5, acetyl L-carnitine is an amino acid that shows some promise in treating diabetic neuropathy. That and another form of L-carnitine, propionyl L-carnitine, have been found to offer potential benefit for diabetic retinopathy.

What Are the Potential Benefits of These Forms of L-Carnitine for Diabetic Retinopathy?

You probably know that electrocardiograms (EKGs) measure the activity of the heart, and electroencephalograms (EEGs) measure brain wave activity. In the same way, electroretinograms measure the activity of the retina. Two different animal studies measured retinal activity in this way. In one study, diabetic rats were tested with and without acetyl L-carnitine (ALC). The ALC supplementation normalized abnormal electroretinograms.[30] In yet another study, a different form of carnitine, propionyl L-carnitine, was found to improve signs of retinal disease in diabetic rats.[31]

Dosage

The oral daily dosage of propionyl L-carnitine or acetyl L-carnitine usually ranges from 500 to 1,000 mg 3 times daily.

Safety Issues

Both forms of L-carnitine discussed here appear to be safe, although extensive formal toxicology tests have not been completed. Safety for young children, pregnant or nursing women, or those with severe liver or kidney disease has not been established.

Magnesium

As we will discuss in chapter 8, people with diabetes are prone to magnesium deficiency. Some researchers theorize that magnesium deficiency contributes to retinopathy in diabetes. However, we have no direct evidence that magnesium supplements can help prevent this condition.

In one study, 71 patients with diabetes who took insulin were divided into two groups, according to the severity of their retinopathy.[32] On average, all the patients had some magnesium deficiency; however, it was more pronounced in the group with the more severe retinopathy.

Dosage and Safety Issues

A reasonable dosage of magnesium is in the range of 200 to 400 mg daily. If diarrhea occurs, the dosage should be reduced. People with kidney disease should avoid doses higher than 100 to 200 mg daily. At this dosage, magnesium is believed to be safe. However, if you suffer from severe kidney or heart disease, do not take magnesium (or any other supplement) except on the advice of a physician.

Vitamin B$_6$

Other researchers have seen a possible link between B$_6$ deficiency and retinopathy, noting an absence of retinopathy in people with diabetes who happened to take B$_6$. Their observations were gathered over periods ranging from 8 months to 28 years.[33] However, as yet we still have no direct evidence that vitamin B$_6$ can help. What we need is a good intervention trial in which some people who have diabetes are given B$_6$ while others are given placebo.

Table 3. Supplements That
May Help Prevent Retinopathy

Bilberry (25% anthocyanosides)	80 to 160 mg 3 times daily
Vitamin C	2 to 4 g daily
Vitamin E	400 to 800 IU daily
Other supplements to consider:	
acetyl L-carnitine, lipoic acid, vitamin B_6, magnesium	

Dosage

A typical safe therapeutic dosage of vitamin B_6 is in the range of 50 to 100 mg daily.

What Are Diabetic Cataracts?

Cataracts result when the lens of the eye gradually becomes opaque, obstructing vision. People with diabetes are prone to develop cataracts earlier and more rapidly than people without diabetes. Cataracts caused by high blood sugar are sometimes referred to as "sugar cataracts."

What Causes Diabetic Cataracts?

In chapter 5 we talked about sorbitol accumulation and how it can contribute to certain complications of diabetes. Cataracts in diabetes are clearly a result of sorbitol buildup in the lens of the eye. Let's briefly review how this happens.

Certain tissues in the body, such as the lens of the eye, do not require insulin for glucose to enter. Glucose can lazily diffuse into cells in the lens if the level of glucose is high in the surrounding fluid. An enzyme called aldose reductase then converts the glucose into a molecule called sorbitol. This molecule cannot escape from the cells of the lens. Water is pulled into the cells after it. This causes the cells to swell, which makes it easier for other molecules, such as sodium, to enter. This swelling and chemical imbalance eventually results in cataracts.

Natural Prevention and Treatment of Diabetic Cataracts

As with most diabetic complications, good blood sugar control is of prime importance in preventing cataracts. Some natural supplements, such as flavonoids, may also be able to help.

Flavonoids

Flavonoids (also called bioflavonoids) are natural constituents found in nearly all plants. Several of these flavonoids may be useful for preventing cataracts in diabetes: quercetin, naringin, and hesperidin.

Quercetin is the most abundant of all the flavonoids. You'll find it in a number of common foods, including onions, apples, tea, berries, and cabbage family vegetables. It is also found in a number of medicinal herbs, including ginkgo, St. John's wort, eucalyptus, and elderberry.

Naringin is a flavonoid found in the fruit, pulp, skin, and flowers of the grapefruit.

Hesperidin is found primarily in oranges and lemons. When you peel citrus fruit, you see that the inner part of the peel has significant amounts of white pulpy stuff. This is where the flavonoids are especially concentrated.

What Are the Potential Benefits of Flavonoids for Diabetic Cataracts?

Certain flavonoids—including quercetin, hesperidin, and naringin—have aldose reductase inhibitor activity.[34, 35]

This means they inhibit the enzyme that converts glucose to sorbitol, making it less likely that sorbitol will build up in the lens of the eye. They are also potent antioxidants.

Aldose reductase inhibitor drugs have been found to prevent diabetic cataracts,[36] although most cause too many side effects to be very useful. If aldose reductase inhibitor drugs can prevent cataracts, and if natural substances such as flavonoids can prevent aldose reductase activity, it is certainly reasonable to suspect that these natural products may help prevent cataracts as well. Unfortunately, we don't have any direct evidence that it works. Test-tube studies have found positive results,[37, 38] but animal studies have been conflicting.[39, 40]

Cataracts in diabetes are clearly a result of sorbitol buildup in the lens of the eye. Some natural substances such as flavonoids may be able to help.

In addition to cataracts, sorbitol buildup in the lens of the eye can contribute to farsightedness (difficulty reading or seeing at close range). If you're farsighted, you might get a secondary benefit from flavonoids, if a rabbit study can be taken as evidence. A study on farsighted diabetic rabbits found flavonoids to significantly improve the farsightedness.[41] The researchers theorized it was the flavonoids' aldose reductase activity that was responsible for the improvement.

Dosage

When taken as a food supplement, the recommended dosage of flavonoids is in the range of 400 to 500 mg 3 times daily.

Safety Issues

Flavonoids are generally considered safe when used in the recommended dosages, although formal safety studies have not been completed.

There has been some controversy about quercetin because it failed to pass what is called the Ames test (a test to see whether a substance causes cell mutation). In addition, an early study on rats implicated quercetin in the development of bladder tumors; however, dozens of subsequent studies have found quercetin to be an anticarcinogen in various test-tube studies of cancer cells including leukemia and tumors of the breast, colon, ovary, uterus, stomach, and lung. Nonetheless, because it may possibly cause mutations, quercetin should be avoided during pregnancy.

A related substance called quercetin chalcone, which is probably better absorbed, did not cause mutations when Ames tested. Its safety during pregnancy has not been evaluated.

No toxicity has been reported for hesperidin. The only known potential problem with naringin is that this substance may interfere with the liver's ability to detoxify certain chemicals. This is actually true of quite a few flavonoid compounds.

However, due to the lack of comprehensive formal safety studies, safety in young children, pregnant or nursing women, or people with severe liver or kidney disease cannot be assured.

Other Natural Substances That May Prevent Cataracts

Several vitamins and other nutrients may prevent cataract formation because they, too, are inhibitors of aldose reductase. Lipoic acid has been found to inhibit aldose reductase.[42] (See chapter 5 for a more complete description of lipoic acid.)

Table 4. Supplements for the Prevention of Diabetic Cataracts

Quercetin (Hesperidin, Naringin)	500 mg 3 times daily
Vitamin C	2 to 4 g daily
Lipoic Acid	200 mg 3 times daily

Several studies have found vitamin C to be a good inhibitor of aldose reductase. In a human study, vitamin C, at doses of 100 to 600 mg daily, was able to normalize accumulations of sorbitol in red blood cells within 30 days.[43] These same researchers found vitamin C to be a good inhibitor of aldose reductase in test-tube studies. Another group of researchers confirmed their findings both in humans and in a test-tube study.[44] See the section earlier in this chapter for a discussion of dosage and safety issues.

A flavonoid from Glycyrrhiza (licorice), known as isoliquiritigenin, has been found in both animal and test-tube studies to be a potent aldose reductase inhibitor.[45] It is not clear how much licorice one would need to consume in order to obtain a therapeutic dose of this flavonoid. Because of the potential for water retention and elevation of blood pressure with long-term use of licorice, the use of other natural aldose reductase inhibitors is advised, unless further studies are done to determine a safe therapeutic dose. For a summary of dosages see table 4.

QUICK REVIEW

- Long-term complications of diabetes include vision problems, particularly retinopathy and cataracts. These complications are mainly due to uncontrolled blood sugar over time.

- The causes of diabetic retinopathy are complex. They are believed to include glycosylation of proteins, free radical damage, increased tendency for the blood to clot, damage to the small blood vessels in the eye, increased leakiness of the blood vessels, and blockage of the vessels by blood clots or thickening of the vessel wall. Whether sorbitol accumulation and elevated homocysteine levels are involved remain controversial issues.

- Maintaining good blood sugar control is the most important aspect of preventing diabetic retinopathy. In addition, several natural supplements may help. Although few human studies have been conducted to determine the effectiveness of vitamin C (2 to 4 g daily), vitamin E (400 to 800 IU daily), and bilberry extract (25% anthocyanosides; 80 to 160 mg 3 times daily), these substances may theoretically help prevent retinopathy.

- People with diabetes are more susceptible to cataracts, caused by sorbitol accumulation in the lens of the eye. Natural substances may prevent this accumulation by inhibiting the enzyme aldose reductase. These include flavonoids such as quercetin (hesperidin, naringin; 500 mg 3 times daily), as well as vitamin C (2 to 4 g daily) and lipoic acid (200 mg 3 times daily).

- **Warning:** Always consult your physician before you give children with diabetes high doses of any vitamin or mineral.

CHAPTER

SEVEN

Heart and Kidney Disease Caused by Diabetes

George had suffered from type 2 diabetes for almost two decades. Despite many attempts at dieting and sporadic bouts of exercise, he was never able to get good control of his blood sugar. When he reached age 60, his doctor gave him some bad news. The blood vessels in and around his heart had dangerous blockages that could lead to heart attack. And, as if that wasn't enough bad news, his doctor told him he was also beginning to show signs of some kidney problems.

Atherosclerosis (the most common type of hardening of the arteries) is the leading cause of death among the population as a whole. However, in diabetics it occurs at an accelerated pace. Atherosclerosis is twice as common in diabetics who have had the disease for at least 10 years as in nondiabetics. In fact, atherosclerosis is the number one cause of early death in type 2 diabetics, and as many as one out of three individuals with type 1 diabetes dies of cardiovascular disease by age 55. The heart attack rate is at least twice as high for both types of diabetes as for nondiabetics.

Blood vessels in other parts of the body besides the heart are affected too, particularly those in the legs and feet. Lack of circulation to the legs and feet can result in tissue death or gangrene, possibly resulting in amputation of toes, feet, and even legs. Among type 1 diabetics, it's estimated that as many as 80 to 85% develop blood vessel disease in the legs after having the disease 20 years. Diabetes also causes kidney damage—as a consequence of accelerated atherosclerosis and other factors.

Dwelling on these risks is not pleasant. But if you have diabetes, it's important that you know about them. The good news is this: You can use many strategies to prevent or slow down the progression of these complications. Control of blood sugar, diet, and exercise are the most important. Besides these, a variety of natural supplements may offer some help.

What Causes Cardiovascular Complications in Diabetes?

Diseases of the heart and blood vessels are more prevalent in diabetics. Why? I'll talk about a number of reasons. Later in this chapter we'll look at natural supplements that may interrupt some of these processes.

As I explained in chapter 6, diabetics are more susceptible to oxidative stress and free radical production than are nondiabetics. In particular, both type 1 and 2 diabetics have a greater susceptibility to oxidation of LDL, the "bad cholesterol."[1] When the LDL cholesterol becomes oxidized, it changes to a size and shape more likely to damage the walls of the blood vessels. This accelerates the development of atherosclerosis. People with diabetes also tend to have higher levels of cholesterol and triglycerides in the blood. These also lead to atherosclerosis.

You will also remember reading in the last chapter that diabetics tend to have blood that forms clots more easily. This factor both directly accelerates atherosclerosis and increases the chance of heart attacks and strokes. Furthermore, in some diabetics the heart muscle may not contract as well. In the last chapter, we talked about proteins with sugars attached called glycosylated proteins. Abnormal amounts of glycosylated proteins have been found in the heart muscle of diabetics. These can contribute to the formation of free radicals, which then cause tissue damage.

Poor circulation in the legs and feet is compounded by the numbness that diabetics often experience in this area, leading to infections of the lower leg, foot, and toes. Because of the numbness, people with diabetes may injure themselves without even being aware of it. Untreated injuries may in turn lead to infection. In addition, repeated undetected trauma can result eventually in ulcers on the feet. Careful and frequent examination of the feet, coupled with impeccable foot hygiene, is an essential part of preventing serious problems.

Diabetic Kidney Disease

Diabetic *nephropathy* is the medical term for kidney disease caused by diabetes. The prevalence of kidney disease is directly related to the length of time the person has had diabetes, and to how well the blood sugar is controlled. The better the blood sugar control, the less the likelihood that kidney problems will develop.

You may remember from the last chapter that the results of a huge, long-term study released in 1998 found that good blood sugar control can significantly reduce damage to the small blood vessels of both the kidneys and the eyes.[2]

The causes of diabetic kidney problems are complicated. Although researchers have found many pieces of the puzzle, science hasn't put them all together yet. Let's examine the puzzle pieces we know about.

Leaky Blood Vessels

The filtration units of the kidneys, called glomeruli, are especially susceptible to damage in diabetes. The ability to filter the blood, excluding certain substances and letting in others, is central to the kidney's functioning. Anything that disrupts this function can lead to problems.

One such disruption occurs when complicated biochemical changes that take place in diabetes cause the capillary membrane to become leaky (just as capillaries in the retina become leaky, as was explained in the last chapter). This allows large molecules like proteins, which are usually barred from entering, to get through.[3] This "open door policy" is why diabetics often have protein in their urine. These proteins themselves may be responsible for some of the kidney damage.

Glycosylated Proteins

It looks like glycosylated proteins are one of the culprits causing biochemical changes that disrupt the capillary membrane and make it leakier.[4] Also, other metabolic abnormalities, too numerous and complicated to describe here, probably contribute to increased capillary leakage in diabetes.

Diminished Filtering Ability

In addition, as with retinopathy, abnormal connective tissue can deposit in the walls of the capillaries in the kidney. The tissue thickens the capillary walls, sometimes blocking them completely. Blocked capillaries keep the kidney from doing its job of filtering the blood. Later stages of diabetic kidney disease are characterized, not by large and small molecules alike passing through too freely, but by just the opposite: the kidneys' diminished ability to filter anything.

Infection
People with diabetes are also more prone to infection of the urinary system. When blood sugar is high, some sugar spills into the urine—to the delight of any bacteria in the neighborhood. The bacteria feeding on the sugar can multiply and cause an infection in the urethra, bladder, or kidneys. Part of the treatment includes controlling blood sugar to decrease the amount of sugar in the urine.

Atherosclerosis
Atherosclerosis, the thickening of blood vessel walls that I described earlier, affects the large vessels leading to the kidneys as well as the small vessels within the kidneys. This further compromises kidney function.

Heart and Kidney: How They Affect Each Other in Diabetes
In diabetes, heart disease and kidney disease are often connected. It's helpful to understand these relationships because many of the natural treatments in this chapter may help prevent both cardiovascular and kidney complications.

The Homocysteine Connection
Diabetics with later stages of kidney disease tend to have high blood levels of homocysteine. Since homocysteine is an amino acid that is eliminated by the kidneys, it is not

Perry's Blood Sugar

Gaining good blood sugar control is often easier said than done. Some people with diabetes, particularly those with type 1 diabetes, have a very difficult time maintaining normal blood sugar no matter how hard they try. Perry was one of those patients—a "brittle diabetic," as people with the most hard-to-control blood sugar are called. Perry organized his life carefully to control his diabetes. He checked his blood sugar many times a day and injected insulin accordingly. He was very careful with his diet, eating much the same food each day. Despite his efforts, however, his blood sugar was often all over the map—bouncing very high, then dipping too low when he overcompensated with too much insulin, then bouncing back up again as his own body's blood-sugar-raising hormones kicked in. The situation was very frustrating for Perry, as well as for me as his doctor.

surprising that people who have difficulty filtering substances—as one would see in late-stage kidney disease—tend to have higher levels in the blood. Unfortunately, high levels of homocysteine appear to accelerate cardiovascular disease. Homocysteine, like the oxidized LDL we talked about above, seems to injure the inside of the blood vessels. The bottom line is this: Kidney disease can cause elevated homocysteine levels, which can in turn result in cardiovascular disease.[5]

The Cholesterol Connection

In addition to elevation of homocysteine, diabetic kidney disease can result in elevated levels of blood fats—cholesterol and triglycerides.[6] These are also risk factors for

Perry has never given up trying to keep his blood sugar under control, and recently he has been more successful. Besides the 50 or so supplements he takes daily, he discovered that combining three types of insulin—the regular, NPH, and newer Humalog—has really helped keep his blood sugar under control most of the time.

I tell this story because it's important for you to understand that controlling blood sugar cannot be taken lightly. The task often takes considerable time and attention—sometimes becoming almost a full-time job. While such control may feel very limiting and be time-consuming, the benefits diabetics reap in years to come may be well worth the time they spend now. By paying careful attention to his blood sugar now, Perry may avoid a kidney transplant or a heart attack in the future.

heart disease. The cholesterol can, in turn, contribute to additional kidney damage, creating a vicious cycle.

Natural Prevention

The old adage, "An ounce of prevention is worth a pound of cure," has never been more true than in the case of diabetic complications in the heart, blood vessels, and kidneys. Once significant damage has occurred in these areas, your only options may be radical measures such as kidney transplant or dialysis for kidney disease.

Why not start preventing these complications early on? To restate what we have said here many times: *Good blood sugar control is key*. It is so important, in fact, that

I'll postpone my discussion of other natural prevention to focus a bit on blood sugar control. (See the sidebar, Perry's Blood Sugar.)

You can go a long way toward accomplishing the goal of good blood sugar control by testing your blood sugar frequently, sticking to your insulin or other medication schedules, and paying careful attention to a good diet (see chapter 2). You may also find the approaches to controlling blood sugar described in chapters 3 and 4 helpful.

In addition to controlling their blood sugar, diabetics might consider taking any of a number of natural supplements that may help prevent serious heart, blood vessel, and kidney damage. Natural treatments include vitamins, such as E and C; minerals, such as selenium and magnesium; essential fatty acids, such as evening primrose oil or fish oil; the amino acid L-carnitine; and plant constituents, such as grape seed extract to decrease capillary leakiness. Taking care to keep homocysteine and cholesterol levels under control is also important. For a more detailed discussion of these treatments in general, see *The Natural Pharmacist Guide to Heart Disease Prevention*. This chapter concentrates on information specifically relevant to diabetes.

Vitamin E—May Offer Many Benefits

Vitamin E is an important nutrient essential for maintaining healthy cell membranes. It is useful for the prevention of cardiovascular disease in particular. Studies have shown that it does several things that are particularly valuable for diabetes. Vitamin E has been found to lower triglycerides, to prevent the oxidation of the bad cholesterol (LDL), to decrease the blood's tendency to clot, and to improve circulation in the kidneys. Let's look at some of the scientific evidence that supports the use of vitamin E in preventing cardiovascular and kidney disease among people with diabetes.

What Is the Scientific Evidence for Vitamin E?

Researchers have studied several effects of vitamin E that may help prevent diabetic heart and kidney disease.

One double-blind study looked at the effect of vitamin E on triglycerides (blood fats that impact heart disease) and glycosylated hemoglobin levels (measures of long-term blood sugar control). Thirty-five type 1 diabetics were given either 100 IU vitamin E daily or placebo for 3 months. Levels of both triglycerides and glycosylated hemoglobin improved significantly in the group on moderately low doses of vitamin E.[7] Animal studies have also found vitamin E to lower triglycerides but not cholesterol in diabetes.[8]

Numerous studies show that vitamin E, as an antioxidant, is capable of preventing oxidation of LDL cholesterol. In one double-blind study, 28 type 1 and 2 diabetics were randomly assigned to receive either 1,200 IU of vitamin E or placebo daily for 8 weeks. In the group receiving vitamin E, LDL was significantly less susceptible to oxidation than in the placebo group.[9] Another double-blind study of 21 type 2 diabetic men found a significant decrease in oxidation of LDL after 10 weeks on high-dose vitamin E (1,600 IU daily) compared to placebo.[10]

> **Numerous studies show that vitamin E is capable of preventing oxidation of LDL cholesterol.**

Although vitamin E may be helpful, it may do no more than good blood sugar control in preventing oxidation of LDL. A study of 15 diabetics on insulin with good blood sugar control found their LDL had the same composition and susceptibility to oxidation as did the LDL of normal, healthy control-group participants.[11] Maintaining good blood sugar control is probably the most important step in preventing blood vessel damage caused by oxidized LDL (although taking vitamin E is easier!).

Vitamin E may have an additional benefit for diabetics: decreasing the stickiness of their platelets, the blood cells responsible for clotting. Diabetics tend to form blood clots more easily because their platelets tend to be stickier—and blood clots, as you know, can cause heart attacks and strokes. Two studies revealed that supplemental vitamin E decreased platelet stickiness in people with diabetes.[12, 13]

The kidney may also benefit from vitamin E. A Russian study of 108 diabetics with damaged blood vessels in their kidneys found vitamin E improved circulation and reduced further free radical–induced kidney damage.[14] Several animal studies have found similar protective effects of vitamin E on the kidneys.[15, 16]

To sum up, vitamin E can help prevent heart and kidney problems by improving circulation, decreasing the oxidized form of the bad cholesterol (LDL), and decreasing the tendency for the blood to form clots.

Dosage

Therapeutic dosage of vitamin E for an adult is in the range of 400 to 1,200 IU daily. Do not, however, take more than 800 IU daily except on the advice of a physician.

Safety Issues

Vitamin E appears to be quite safe, even when taken in very high doses. Even so, it does present a few potential risks. Because vitamin E has the potential to thin the blood, talk with your doctor before using it with other blood thinning medications or supplements, such as Coumadin (warfarin), heparin, or aspirin. It is also at least remotely possible that vitamin E could interact with natural substances that have a mild blood thinning effect, such as garlic and ginkgo. Also, some researchers have found vitamin E to elevate already high blood pressure in certain people. If you have high blood pressure, monitor it when you begin supplementing with vitamin E.

Selenium

Selenium is an important antioxidant mineral that appears to team up with vitamin E in the body. Like vitamin E, the beneficial effects of selenium seem to be related to its antioxidant and blood thinning effects. Before we can say with any certainty that selenium supplements will help people with diabetes, however, further research must be done. In a group of type 1 diabetics, those with low selenium in their red blood cells also had "thicker" blood.[17] This study, although promising, does not tell us that taking additional selenium will "thin" the blood.

An animal study found selenium to delay the onset of injury to the kidneys caused by diabetes.[18] It appeared to offer even more protection when combined with vitamin E.

Dosage

Therapeutic dose of selenium is in the range of 100 to 200 mcg daily.

Safety Issues

Selenium can be toxic if taken in doses above about 500 mcg. Before supplementing with selenium, examine your multiple vitamin–mineral supplements to be sure you are not already getting enough of this mineral. Maximum safe doses for young children, pregnant or nursing women, or those with severe liver or kidney disease have not been determined.

Essential Fatty Acids

A number of important nutritional fats—essential fatty acids—are necessary for good health. They may also be important in preventing and treating problems associated with diabetes. Study results, however, have been conflicting. Let's attempt to sort truth from fiction. We'll look separately at fish oils and vegetable oils.

In reporting on these studies, I'll be referring to various measurements of cholesterol and triglycerides. Here's a quick review to help you keep the facts straight in your mind:

- Cholesterol occurs as HDL and LDL,
  among other types.
- HDL is good.
- LDL is bad.
- Total cholesterol includes all types. Usually something that raises total cholesterol is bad.
- Triglycerides are often measured along with cholesterol. They are bad, although not as bad as LDL and total cholesterol.

Fish Oil

Fish oil high in the essential fatty acids EPA and DHA appears to provide some protection from cardiovascular disease by decreasing the bad fats in the blood and increasing the good ones. It appears to be more effective at reducing triglycerides than cholesterol. Let's look at what researchers have found.

What's the Scientific Evidence for
Essential Fatty Acids?

In a small uncontrolled study, 8 type 2 diabetics were given 8 g omega-3 fatty acids daily. After 2 months they had good news: their average total triglycerides went down 33%. Total cholesterol also decreased by 11%, but LDL and HDL were unchanged.[19]

The next two studies compared fish oil with either olive or flaxseed oil. A double-blind study on 18 people with type 1 diabetes compared cod liver oil (high in omega-3 oils) with olive oil (devoid of omega-3 oils), and found cod liver oil to decrease triglycerides and have no effect on the LDL cholesterol.[20] The good guy, the HDL cholesterol, was increased, but total cholesterol showed no significant change.

Another study comparing fish oil with flaxseed oil found similar results.[21] A significant decrease in triglycerides was found in the fish oil but not the flaxseed oil group. This may be because there is some indication that diabetics can not convert the essential fatty acids in the flaxseed oil to important substances needed to lower triglycerides.[22]

The bottom line is this: Fish oil seems to lower triglycerides, but its effects on LDL, HDL, and total cholesterol levels are not consistent in diabetes.

Fish oil may also help by making the red blood cell membrane more flexible. The more flexible the red blood cell, the more easily it passes through the tiny capillaries. In a controlled study, diabetics and healthy controls both received 2.7 g daily of sardine oil (high in omega 3 fatty acids).[23] At the beginning of the study, the red blood cells in the diabetic group were significantly less flexible. After 4 weeks the flexibility increased in both groups, and differences between the two groups disappeared. The flexibility stayed high during the entire 8 weeks of the study. This has potential importance for diabetic kidney disease. For proper kidney function, red blood cells must be able to pass through the tiny capillaries of the kidneys.

Dosage

Fish oil should be taken in a dose that supplies 3 g daily of omega-3 fatty acids. The total amount of fish oil necessary to supply this varies with the product. Fish high in omega-3 fatty acids include salmon, sardines, mackerel, haddock, and herring. The liver of cod (hence cod liver oil) is also high in omega-3 fatty acids; however, it also includes enough vitamin A and D to be potentially dangerous (see Safety Issues).

Use caution with cod liver oil, because it is very high in vitamins A and D—two vitamins we store in our bodies.

Safety Issues

Fish oil generally appears to be safe. However, one study caused some alarm by suggesting that fish oil can raise LDL cholesterol in people with diabetes.[24] However, the dose used (15 g daily) was much higher than the dosage normally recommended (3 g daily). Some concerns exist that excessive intake of fish oil can provide enough extra calories to raise blood sugar levels. To be on the safe side, be sure you closely evaluate your blood sugar and cholesterol when you supplement with fish oil.

In addition, you should use caution with cod liver oil, because it is very high in vitamins A and D—two vitamins we store in our bodies. Since most people get plenty of these vitamins from other sources, they may actually get a toxic dose when supplementing with cod liver oil. This is a particular risk for pregnant women.

Fish oil also has some potential to oxidize, turning into unhealthy fats. The addition of vitamin E may help prevent this transformation.[25]

Omega-6 Fatty Acids—
May Help Prevent Heart Disease

You may remember that in chapter 5 we said that GLA—an omega-6 fatty acid from evening primrose oil, black currant oil, or borage oil—could be helpful in treating diabetic neuropathy. Some of these essential fatty acids may also have some benefit in preventing heart disease in diabetes.

One interesting study suggests that linoleic acid, another omega-6 fatty acid found in safflower and most other vegetable oils, may make a difference in preventing diabetic heart disease.[26]

This study looked at 102 people newly diagnosed with diabetes, half of whom received a diet enriched with linoleic acid. After 5 years, people on the special diet had fewer cardiovascular problems than did the remaining subjects, who remained on a standard Western diet. Three men on the Western diet died of a heart attack during the study, whereas none of the participants on the high linoleic acid diet died. Of those who survived the full 5 years of the study, 4% of the women and 6% of the men in the linoleic acid group suffered heart damage from decreased oxygen to the heart muscle. In contrast, 16% of the women and 22% of the men in the Western diet group suffered such heart damage.

The body converts linoleic acid to GLA. However, you may remember from chapter 5 that people with diabetes may have trouble carrying out this conversion. Did the people taking linoleic acid in this study improve because they managed to convert it to GLA? If so, they might do even better with GLA supplements than with linoleic acid. Unfortunately, while GLA has been tested and found to benefit diabetics with neuropathy, we still need research in the area of cardiovascular disease in diabetes.

Dosage

If you use GLA, take about 3 g daily. If you want to include vegetable oils in your diet, try 1 to 2 tablespoons cold-pressed oil daily as a salad dressing.

Safety Issues

Polyunsaturated oils, such as safflower oil, can result in the formation of free radicals, particularly if you heat them. As with fish oils, you are well advised to take them along with vitamin E and other antioxidants.

Lowering Homocysteine Levels

Recent studies suggest that supplemental folic acid, B_{12}, and vitamin B_6 can lower homocysteine levels in nondiabetics (see *The Natural Pharmacist Guide to Heart Disease Prevention* for more information). It seems likely that the same supplements would be helpful in people with diabetes, but this has not been proven.

Vitamin C

Some evidence suggests that vitamin C may be helpful in decreasing cholesterol. In a double-blind trial, 48 people with type 2 diabetes who had high cholesterol were given 500 mg of vitamin C or placebo daily for 1 year.[27] The placebo group showed no change, but 60% of the vitamin C group experienced a 40% reduction in cholesterol levels and smaller decreases in triglyceride levels.

Dosage and Safety Issues

Please refer to chapter 8 for dosage and safety information for vitamin C.

L-Carnitine

L-carnitine is an amino acid found in high concentrations in muscles, especially in the heart. Many studies have focused on its use in prevention and treatment of heart problems, not necessarily related to diabetes. That topic is beyond the scope of this book.

What's the Scientific Evidence for L-Carnitine?

In this section I'll briefly touch on a couple of studies on L-carnitine in kidney disease. These studies were performed with subjects who were on kidney dialysis for a variety of reasons, not necessarily diabetes. One study showed that L-carnitine may be helpful for patients on kidney dialysis. Dialysis patients frequently have a deficiency of this important amino acid. In addition, they often experience muscle weakness, possibly due to this deficiency. L-carnitine, given in a fairly small dose of 500 mg daily, improved the symptoms of muscle weakness in 20 of the 30 patients after 12 weeks.[28]

In another study, 1,000 mg of L-carnitine or placebo was given to 101 patients before and after dialysis for either 3 or 6 months. In the 3-month group, L-carnitine supplementation improved patients' energy and their perception of the quality of their life. In the 6-month group, the same phenomena occurred early on but was not sustained throughout the study.[29]

Dosage

Dosage is in the range of 500 to 1,000 mg 3 times daily (dosages used in the above studies were somewhat less). No formal safety studies have been done. Studies on pregnant animals showed that no harm to the fetus resulted.

Minor side effects include stomach upset and body odor. Researchers also noted neurological symptoms in people with kidney impairment using the DL rather than the L form of carnitine.[30] People with kidney impairment should take L-carnitine (and all other supplements) only with medical supervision.

Safety in young children, pregnant or nursing women, or people with severe liver disease has not been established.

Grape Seed Extract

Oligomeric proanthocyanidins—also called OPCs or PCOs—are a component of certain plants. The most common commercial source of this supplement, which may be helpful for diabetic kidney disease, is grape seeds.

What's the Scientific Evidence for OPCs?

Like bilberry (see chapter 6), OPCs appear to decrease the leakiness and fragility of capillaries, according to a study of people with diabetes or high blood pressure.[31] In this double-blind and placebo-controlled study, participants took 150 mg daily. As we have discussed previously in this chapter, decreasing the leakiness and fragility of capillaries is important for the function of the kidneys. However, we don't have any good evidence yet that OPCs can prevent or treat diabetic kidney disease.

Dosage

The usual dosage of grape seed extract is in the range of 100 to 300 mg daily.

Safety Issues

Detailed toxicological studies have found grape seed extract in the recommended dosages to be very safe.[32] However, maximum safe dosages in young children, pregnant or nursing women, or those with severe liver or kidney disease have not been established.

Garlic

Garlic has been extensively studied in nondiabetics for its benefits in lowering cholesterol and preventing or reversing atherosclerosis by other means. However, it has not been studied in diabetics specifically. A typical dose is 900 mg daily of garlic powder standardized to contain 1.3% alliin. Because garlic "thins" the blood, it should not be combined with Coumadin (warfarin), heparin, or perhaps even aspirin, except on a physician's advice. There is also at least a theoretical possibility that garlic might interact with natural substances that thin the blood slightly, such as ginkgo and high-dose vitamin E. See *The Natural Pharmacist Guide to Garlic and Cholesterol* for more information.

Taurine

Taurine is an important amino acid found in high concentrations in the heart. A study found 39 people with type 1 diabetes to have deficient blood levels of taurine when compared to 34 controls who had the same daily protein intake.[33] Oral supplementation of 1.5 g daily for 90 days corrected the deficiency and also led to decreased platelet stickiness in the diabetic group. Taurine may help prevent atherosclerosis or its consequences, but there is no direct evidence. In one study in diabetic rats, taurine decreased protein in the urine (a sign of impaired kidney function) by 50%.[34]

The typical dosage of taurine is in the range of 1 to 3 g daily. The maximum safe dose of taurine in young children, pregnant or nursing women, or those with severe liver or kidney disease has not been established.

Magnesium

Magnesium is an important mineral for maintaining a healthy heart. Since diabetics tend to be deficient in magnesium, additional supplementation for the prevention of diabetes-induced heart and blood vessel problems may be indicated.[35]

Dosage and Safety Issues

Individuals with severe heart disease should not take magnesium (or any other supplement) except on physician advice. Please refer to chapter 8 for dosage and additional safety recommendations.

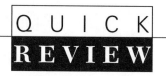

- Heart and kidney diseases are the leading causes of death among diabetics. Specific causes of each are complex. Good blood sugar control is the most important factor in preventing these devastating complications. The best ways to control blood sugar include careful testing, proper administration of medications, and attention to diet. Also consider a good comprehensive supplement program for blood sugar control (discussed in chapters 3 and 4).

- Vitamins That May Help Prevent Diabetic Cardiovascular and Kidney Problems

    Vitamin E: Decreases LDL oxidation, "thins" the blood, decreases glycosylated proteins, lowers triglycerides (400 to 800 IU daily). Do not combine with other blood thinners, such as Coumadin (warfarin), heparin, or aspirin, except on physician's advice.

    Vitamin C: Increases capillary strength, decreases capillary leakiness, improves collagen formation in the lining of blood vessels, lowers cholesterol (1 to 4 g daily).

- Minerals that may help prevent heart and kidney problems:

    Selenium: Antioxidant, blood thinner, protects the kidneys from damage in animal studies (100 to 200 mcg daily).

    Magnesium: Important mineral for healthy heart muscle function; dilates blood vessels to lower blood pressure; often deficient in diabetics (200 to 400 mg daily).

    Individuals with severe heart or kidney disease should not take magnesium (or any other supplement) except with physician's advice.

- Essential fatty acids that may help prevent heart and kidney problems:

    Fish oils: Lower triglycerides, reduce protein leakage by the kidneys, improve red blood cell flexibility (3 g daily or eat coldwater fish listed above 3 or more times a week).

    Omega-6 fatty acids: Lower bad cholesterol (LDL), increase the good cholesterol (HDL). GLA, EPO, borage, black currant oil (3 g daily); cold-pressed oils such as safflower (1 to 2 tablespoons daily).

- Amino acids that may help prevent heart and kidney problems:

    L-carnitine: Improves muscle weakness and energy in dialysis patients, enhances heart function, lowers triglycerides (500 to 1,000 mg 3 times daily).

    Taurine: Important amino acid for proper heart function, decreases protein in the urine in animal studies, reduces platelet stickiness (1 to 3 g daily).

- Herbs that may help prevent heart and kidney problems:

    Oligomeric proanthocyanidins (OPC, PCO, pycnogenol, grape seed extract): Decrease capillary leakiness and fragility; antioxidant (100 to 300 mg daily).

Garlic: Reduces cholesterol levels and atherosclerosis (900 mg daily of garlic powder standardized to contain 1.3% alliin). Because garlic "thins" the blood, it should not be combined with other blood thinning agents such as Coumadin (warfarin), heparin, or aspirin, except on physician's advice.

- Be sure to refer to the chapter for safety issues regarding these supplements.

Diabetes and
Nutritional Deficiencies

I n chapters 3 through 7 we explored various vitamins, minerals, and herbs that might help control blood sugar, as well as help prevent diabetic complications. Here the focus is different. Rather than discuss how nutrients in high doses can help control specific symptoms, I instead talk about making sure you get the nutrients you need for good general health. Occasionally I'll mention symptoms linked to a particular nutrient deficiency, but emphasize maintaining good health overall. All people are healthier when they have all the nutrients they need, and people with diabetes are no exception. Being malnourished simply isn't a good idea.

Please note that a person with diabetes who has severe kidney disease needs to exert extra caution, even with something as wholesome as vitamins. Kidney disease interferes with the processing of all nutrients. If you have severe kidney disease, do not take any of the supplements described in this chapter except on a doctor's recommendation.

Bob's Story

Bob, age 48, had been diagnosed with type 2 diabetes 7 years previously. Since then he'd forced himself to live without his two favorite foods: French fries and eggs Benedict. But, while he avoided the worst dietary culprits, he did not like most vegetables so did not eat nearly enough of them. Concerned that he might be lacking in important nutrients, he began taking a daily multivitamin/mineral supplement. He suspected it didn't fully replace a big plate of broccoli, but it was easier on his taste buds. Bob's doctor

Like most diseases, diabetes can result in an increased need for certain vitamins and minerals. Individuals with diabetes who experience poor blood sugar control and increased urination are prone to lose important vitamins and minerals in the urine, such as vitamin C. Some of the medications used to treat diabetes can also promote deficiencies—for example, some oral diabetes drugs can cause poor absorption of B_{12}. The sidebar, Why Does Diabetes Cause Nutritional Deficiencies? lists some of the many reasons you may be nutrient deficient if you have diabetes.

It's important to remember that being diabetic doesn't mean you *will* have serious deficiencies. Some researchers in Germany examined vitamin levels in 119 individuals with diabetes and found that, in general, all study participants were well supplied with vitamins B_1, B_2, and E. They found levels of B_6 and B_{12} to be occasionally low.[1]

The best solution, of course, is to obtain all the nutrients you need by eating a good diet. But because of the increased nutrient demands in the disease, it may be prudent for people with diabetes to take a good quality, high-potency multiple vitamin/mineral.

felt this was a wise move. Besides helping protect Bob from his dietary lapses, the supplement also gave him the extra nutrients he might need as a person with diabetes. The doctor explained that Bob might be losing some nutrients in his urine, and that his medication—metformin—might be interfering with absorption as well. They both hoped the supplement would supply him with the nutrients he needed and keep him healthier overall.

Common Nutrient Deficiencies in Diabetes

Both diabetes and the medications used to treat it can cause people with diabetes to fall short of various nutrients. If you can make up for these deficiencies, either through diet or supplementation, you are likely to become a healthier person overall. Furthermore, certain nutrient deficiencies may actually increase the severity of diabetes and its complications. For example, vitamin E deficiency may contribute to retinopathy, since individuals with diabetes, particularly those with retinopathy appear to have lower than normal vitamin E levels, as we discussed in chapter 6. Diabetics may also have an increased risk of neuropathy with a vitamin B_6 deficiency, since such a deficiency can cause neuropathy even in people without diabetes. Now, let's look at the specific deficiencies to which those with diabetes are prone. First we'll look at the best-documented deficiency: magnesium. Then we'll turn to other vitamins and minerals. For a listing of food sources for some common deficiencies see table 5.

Magnesium

Magnesium deficiency is the most common mineral deficiency in insulin-dependent diabetes.[2] Diabetes is the most common disease contributing to this deficiency[3] and it is more common in diabetics than in the general population.[4] There are many proposed causes for magnesium deficiency in diabetes, which involve complicated changes in the metabolism of people with diabetes; but that discussion is beyond the scope of this book.

Being deficient in any mineral is not a good idea; for this reason alone, those with diabetes should make sure to get enough magnesium. You can increase the amount of magnesium in your diet by eating foods such as green leafy vegetables and whole grains (see table 5 for a more complete list). If you'd prefer to take a magnesium supplement, a dosage of 300 to 400 mg daily is recommended. If you find this causes diarrhea, cut back.

Besides contributing to overall malnutrition, magnesium deficiency may be specifically associated with certain complications of diabetes. This was the focus of a study involving 71 individuals with diabetes on insulin, all of whom had some degree of retinopathy.[5] Those with the most severe retinopathy were in one group, and those having less severe retinopathy were in another group. Low magnesium levels were found in both groups, but the deficiency was most pronounced in the group with the most severe retinopathy.

Certain nutrient deficiencies may increase the likelihood or severity of diabetes and its complications.

Vitamin C

People with diabetes on insulin were found to be low in vitamin C, even though they consumed

Why Does Diabetes Cause Nutritional Deficiencies?

■ People with diabetes seem to absorb certain nutrients less well than the general population.

■ Some vitamins, such as vitamin C, require insulin to enter most cells. A low level of insulin may result in a low level of vitamin C inside the cells.

■ People with diabetes may have problems converting a particular vitamin to its active form, or may tend to convert a particular vitamin, such as vitamin C, to a less active form.

■ Certain drugs for diabetes may promote deficiencies in vitamins such as B_{12}, perhaps by interfering with absorption.

seemingly adequate amounts in their diets.[6] In experiments on animals with diabetes, researchers found that high blood sugar levels caused increased loss of vitamin C in the urine.[7] Again, it is not wise to be deficient in an essential nutrient. Those with diabetes should probably pay extra attention to getting enough vitamin C daily.

Research suggests that vitamin C deficiency might be caused by high blood sugar increasing the conversion of vitamin C to its undesirable oxidized form, dehydroascorbic acid.[8]

Even when one has adequate vitamin C in the blood, evidence suggests that high blood sugar may inhibit its uptake by the cells.[9] Vitamin C (just like sugar) needs insulin to get into most cells; therefore, if the blood sugar is high, that means there is not enough insulin on board, either for the sugar or the vitamin C to get into the cells.

You can increase the amount of vitamin C in your diet by eating foods such as citrus fruits, broccoli, tomatoes, and many other fruits and vegetables, or by taking a vitamin C supplement of 500 mg or more (see table 5).

Certain supplements, such as vitamin E and lipoic acid, can convert dehydroascorbic acid back to ascorbic acid or "the good form of vitamin C." If you are diabetic, you might consider taking some vitamin E and/or lipoic acid with it. (Besides neutralizing dehydroascorbic acid, both vitamin E and lipoic acid may help prevent certain diabetic complications, as we discussed in the last three chapters.)

Vitamin B_{12} (Cobalamin)

Two drugs taken orally to reduce blood sugar, metformin and phenformin, have been found to promote a B_{12} deficiency, apparently by interfering with absorption.[10] Testing for B_{12} deficiency is easy, unlike for some of the other nutrients discussed in this chapter. People with diabetes who take metformin or phenformin to reduce blood sugar should consider having their B_{12} levels checked to see whether they need extra B_{12}. A deficiency of this vitamin can lead to nerve damage, a risk diabetics already face. Because B_{12} is found in substantial amounts only in animal products, vegetarians may be at particular risk. A B_{12} supplement containing 500 to 1,000 mcg B_{12} is recommended. Cheese, eggs, and other animal foods contain good amounts of vitamin B_{12}.

Vitamin A

Evidence suggests that vitamin A levels are lower in diabetics than in nondiabetics. A couple theories suggest why this might occur.

One theory is that people with diabetes may have difficulty accessing their vitamin A, which is stored in the liver.[11, 12] Evidence suggests that people with type 1 but not type 2 diabetes may be deficient in a substance called "retinol binding protein," which carries vitamin A from the liver to places where it is needed, such as to the retina. This may be particularly true for those who have difficulty controlling their blood sugar.

Another theory is based on the fact that we get much of our vitamin A by eating foods rich in beta-carotene, which gets converted to vitamin A in our bodies. Beta-carotene is found widely in the yellow pigments of fruits and vegetables (carrots, squash, and melons, for example). People with diabetes may not be very efficient at converting beta-carotene to vitamin A.

Only a few foods contain pre-formed vitamin A, primarily the livers of fish and other animals. If you have diabetes, especially if you are a vegetarian, you should probably take a vitamin A supplement, or a multiple vitamin containing vitamin A rather than beta-carotene. Be sure to check how much vitamin A you are getting in all your supplements, and don't exceed the recommended levels. Excess vitamin A can cause liver damage. This is true for everyone, but it may be even more important for people with diabetes, since, as mentioned above, they may have a particularly hard time getting vitamin A out of the liver. However, this also means that taking extra vitamin A even in appropriate amounts may not be helpful, if the vitamin A just stays in the liver. The best way to improve vitamin A levels may be to ensure good blood sugar control.

Warning: Be careful not to overdo vitamin A supplements, since it's fairly easy to take too much.

A recommended dosage of vitamin A is 5,000 IU daily.

Vitamin E

People with diabetes may have an increased requirement for vitamin E, making a deficiency more likely.[13] However, some of the same researchers who studied vitamin A levels in diabetes found no difference in vitamin E levels between diabetics and nondiabetics.[14] As we discussed in chapters 5, 6, and 7, taking vitamin E even if you don't have a deficiency of the vitamin may be worthwhile. Vitamin E is a potent antioxidant, and may help prevent retinopathy, neuropathy, cardiovascular, and kidney complications.

Vitamin E is a potent antioxidant, and may help prevent retinopathy, neuropathy, and cardiovascular and kidney complications.

A typical dosage for vitamin E is in the range of 400 to 800 IU daily. However, if taken in large doses along with drugs that "thin" the blood, such as Coumadin (warfarin), heparin, or aspirin, vitamin E may pose a risk of bleeding. If you are taking one of these medications, consult with your physician before you add vitamin E supplements to your regimen. There is also at least a slight possibility that vitamin E could interact with natural products that thin the blood, such as garlic or ginkgo.

Biotin

Some people with diabetes appear to have either a deficiency of or an inability to properly utilize the B vitamin biotin, found in cooked egg yolks, some fish, and other foods listed in table 5. (Please note, however, that eating raw egg whites can actually rob your body of biotin.) This deficiency is important because low levels of biotin may contribute to peripheral neuropathy—nerve damage in the arms, legs, and feet.[15] You may want to supplement with 300 mcg daily. As described in chapter 3, much higher doses (in the range of 16 mg daily) are sometimes recommended to lower blood sugar.

Chromium

As described in chapter 3, chromium supplements may be helpful for people with diabetes. It is natural to reason from this that chromium deficiency is common in diabetics, but we have no direct evidence that this is the case. One problem is that the normal level of chromium in the blood is so minute that it's extremely difficult to measure reliably. See chapter 3 for dosage recommendations.

Other Minerals

Weak evidence suggests that people with diabetes may be deficient in manganese[16] and phosphorus.[17] They may also be deficient in zinc, but the evidence is somewhat contradictory. A few studies found diabetics to be deficient in zinc when compared to nondiabetics.[18, 19] However, other studies found an elevated level of zinc in the blood of people with diabetes, perhaps because of their inability to store it properly in the cells.[20]

Evidence shows that potassium may be depleted in diabetes;[21, 22] however, potassium supplementation may not be a good idea. People with diabetes sometimes have a decreased ability to eliminate this mineral from the body via the kidneys, which means they might accumulate dangerously high levels of potassium.[23, 24]

Warning: Do *not* supplement potassium (other than the 100 mg or so you might get from a multiple vitamin) without the supervision of your doctor, who can easily test your potassium levels periodically.

Other Common Nutrient Deficiencies

As you are probably beginning to see, diabetes can have a profound effect on the body's metabolism. It should be no surprise that people with diabetes may be deficient in other nutrients besides vitamins and minerals.

Table 5. Food Sources of Some Common Nutrient Deficiencies in Diabetes

Nutrient	Food Sources
Vitamin A	liver, cod liver oil
Vitamin B_1	beans, brown rice, egg yolks, meat, fish, nuts, asparagus, broccoli, oats
Vitamin B_2	beans, cheese, eggs, fish, poultry, spinach, yogurt
Vitamin B_6	brewer's yeast, carrots, chicken, eggs, fish, meat, peas, spinach, walnuts, wheat germ
Vitamin B_{12}	only found in animal products: blue cheese, cheese, clams, eggs, herring, kidney, liver, mackerel, and all other animal products
Biotin	cooked egg yolk, salt-water fish, meat, milk, poultry, soybeans, whole grains, yeast (avoid raw egg whites as they may cause a deficiency)
Vitamin C	citrus fruits (oranges, grapefruit, lemons), strawberries, mangos, papayas, pineapple, bell peppers, broccoli, tomatoes, green leafy vegetables (spinach, collard greens, Swiss chard, turnip greens, beet greens)
Vitamin E	cold-pressed vegetable oils, whole grains, dark green leafy vegetables, nuts, seeds, beans, eggs, wheat germ, liver
CoQ_{10}	mackerel, salmon, sardines, muscle meat, beef or chicken heart
Chromium	brewer's yeast, brown rice, cheese, mushrooms, corn, chicken, dried beans
Magnesium	green leafy vegetables, whole grains, dairy products, fish, tofu, brown rice, millet, apples, apricots, bananas, meat
Manganese	blueberries, avocados, nuts, seeds, seaweed, whole grains, egg yolks, green leafy vegetables
Phosphorus	deficiency rare as it is found in most foods including soda pop, meat, food additives, brewer's yeast, corn, dairy products, eggs

(continues)

Nutrient	Food Sources
Potassium	winter squash, bananas, potatoes, fish, apricots, avocados, blackstrap molasses, brewer's yeast, dried fruit, yams
Zinc	oysters, pumpkin seeds, soybeans, egg yolks, fish, meat, poultry, liver, lima beans

Essential Fatty Acids

Individuals with diabetes may be deficient in important essential fatty acids (EFAs).[25, 26] Just as for vitamins and minerals, you don't want to be short on EFAs either.

A good supplemental dose is 3 g daily of a combination of fish oil and GLA from borage, black currant, or evening primrose oil.

CoEnzyme Q_{10} (CoQ$_{10}$)

CoEnzyme Q_{10}, popularly known as CoQ_{10}, is a vitamin-like substance that plays a central role in the body's capacity to make energy from food. Since we produce it in our bodies, it is not officially a vitamin. However, one group of researchers observed that 20% of people with diabetes on oral blood sugar–lowering medications were deficient in this important nutrient.[27] The medications they found contributing to a deficiency were tolazamide, a member of the sulfonylurea group; and phenformin, from the biguanide group. Supplementation with CoQ_{10} at a dose of 30 to 60 mg daily may be advisable. CoQ_{10} appears to be a very safe substance.

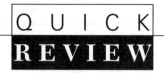

- Many researchers have found that people with diabetes tend to be deficient in certain nutrients, particularly vitamins and minerals. Causes for a deficiency include an increased nutrient requirement, poor absorption, increased loss via the kidneys, impairment of metabolism, and certain anti-diabetic medications.

- You can help yourself maintain good general health by getting enough of all the nutrients you need.

- People with kidney disease should take supplements only under a physician's guidance.

- Taking a multivitamin and mineral supplement may be a simple way of ensuring that you are getting enough of the nutrients you need.

- Be aware of the total amount you are taking of each nutrient in your multivitamin before adding additional supplements. Certain vitamins (such as vitamin A) can be toxic in large doses, and others may interact with medications. Take large doses only under the supervision of your doctor.

- Magnesium is probably the most significant deficiency among people with diabetes. It's worth paying particular attention to this, as magnesium deficiency may contribute to some diabetic complications such as retinopathy.

  You can increase the amount of magnesium in your diet by eating foods such as green leafy vegetables and whole grains (see table 5 for a more complete list).

If you'd prefer to take a magnesium supplement, a dosage of 300 to 400 mg daily is recommended.

- Other nutrients that have been documented to be deficient in some people with diabetes include vitamins C, A, and B_{12}. An easy blood test will show whether you are low in B_{12}.

    Vitamin C: Take a vitamin C supplement of 500 mg or more, or increase the amount of vitamin C in your diet by eating foods such as citrus fruits, broccoli, tomatoes, and many other fruits and vegetables (see table 5).

    Vitamin B_{12}: A B_{12} supplement containing 500 to 1,000 mcg B_{12} is recommended. Cheese, eggs, and other animal foods contain good amounts of vitamin B_{12}.

- Taking large doses of vitamin A to counteract a deficiency may not be helpful because the problem may be difficulty accessing the vitamin A stored in the liver. Taking more may add to toxic accumulation. Better blood sugar control is probably the key.

    Vitamin A: 5,000 IU daily, however, see chapter for additional safety warnings.

- Evidence of deficiencies in vitamin E, biotin, and CoQ_{10} glutathione is relatively weak.

- Studies on zinc and potassium have been inconsistent, with some finding a deficiency in people with diabetes and others reporting an excess in this population.

- No one has been able to determine whether people with diabetes tend to be deficient in chromium because reliable tests are not available.

Preventing Diabetes Naturally

W e've spent most of this book talking about natural
approaches to managing diabetes and preventing
complications in people who already have the disease. In this chapter, I'll discuss a subject that's potentially
even more important: actual prevention of diabetes. Exciting research is being conducted on prevention of both
type 1 and type 2 diabetes. Since the causes of the two
types differ, approaches to their prevention differ as well.
I'll talk about what's known regarding natural prevention
of each type.

Is It Possible to Prevent Type 1 Diabetes?

If you have a child with type 1 diabetes, or if you have it
yourself, you've probably spent some time wondering
about prevention. You may remember from chapter 1 that
type 1 diabetes arises in genetically susceptible people.

Diabetes is significantly more likely to develop in a person with a family history of the disease. As we shall see below, there are other possible ways to find out whether your child is at greater than average risk.

But, most importantly, you may be able to do something about preventing diabetes. This chapter will discuss the evidence for taking steps to prevent type 1 diabetes. It will also briefly touch on preventing type 2 diabetes, which presents very different issues.

Who's at Risk for Type 1 Diabetes?

A general rule in medicine states that prevention should be targeted at those most at risk. For some diseases, such as heart disease, everyone is at risk; and taking some steps to prevent it makes sense for everyone. But the types of prevention practitioners recommend for the population at large are usually fairly general—lifestyle issues such as increasing exercise and improving diet. When you get into taking medications, however, doctors ordinarily want to focus a bit closer. Because all drugs can cause side effects, you want to make sure that the disease risk is worth the treatment risk.

Focusing on certain high-risk people is even more important when a relatively rare disease such as type 1 diabetes is involved. Even though the steps described in this chapter are fairly benign, you may wish to have a special reason to believe that your child is at increased risk for diabetes before taking them. But how do you know what the odds are that your healthy 2 year old may develop diabetes by age 20?

On average, people with an immediate relative (parent, sibling, or child) with diabetes have a 10% chance of developing type 1 diabetes at some point in their lives. New screening tests can help you determine whether your

Vivian's Story

Vivian's oldest daughter, Theresa, was diagnosed with diabetes at age 9. She'd been vomiting, and Vivian took her to the doctor, who diagnosed flu. After 3 days of 7-Up, Theresa became stuporous. Terrified, Vivian rushed her to the emergency room. It turned out that her daughter had diabetes, and had developed diabetic ketoacidosis. Fortunately, insulin and intravenous fluids restored the balance, and Theresa was feeling better in a couple of days. Mother and daughter learned all they could about the disease, and Theresa's diabetes stayed under good control with daily insulin injections.

Several years later, Vivian gave birth to another daughter. A happy, laughing baby, Cecilia took her bottle eagerly and seemed to thrive. When Cecilia was 8 years old, however, Vivian noticed that she seemed to be drinking a lot and using the restroom too often. Suspicious, she tested Cecilia's blood sugar, using a disposable lancet from Theresa's supply.

child is at high risk. These tests measure levels of anti-pancreas antibodies. The most commonly used is the islet cell antibody (ICA) test. Risk of developing diabetes may increase to as much as 62% if a child has high levels of ICA antibodies. If certain other antibodies are also high, their risk may increase to nearly 90%, according to some researchers.[1]

If your child is at increased risk, you may wish to use one or both of the methods described below, even though they haven't been conclusively proven effective at this time. Older individuals who are at high risk for diabetes may also use the second method.

Sure enough: the reading was over 300! The doctor praised Vivian's quick thinking. She'd been alert to her child's increased thirst and urination, and picked up the diabetes before it led to a trip to the emergency room.

Vivian appreciated the doctor's praise, but wondered— was there some way she could have prevented Cecilia's diabetes? She knew what the doctor would say: Cecilia's heredity made her more susceptible than the average child, and nobody knows what triggers the disease. She knew, too, that she shouldn't feel guilty—still, she couldn't help thinking about it. Perhaps she should have breastfed longer, she thought. She even irrationally beat herself up about taking her daughter to the babysitter when Cecilia was so young. Above all, she wished the experts knew more about prevention, because she had recently remarried and was planning to have another child.

Breastfeeding Versus Formula: The Cow's Milk Connection

Scientists are studying a possible link between drinking cow's milk in infancy and developing type 1 diabetes. This may seem hard to believe, since we are taught that "everybody needs milk." Sure, everybody needs milk. Humans need human milk, cows need cow's milk, cats need cat's milk, and so on—at least as babies. It is drinking the milk of another species that may cause problems. Why? Animal milk contains proteins that are foreign to the human body and may trigger harmful immune responses.

To understand what's behind this, we'll review a bit of our discussion from chapter 1. Type 1 diabetes is an auto-immune disease—that is, a disease in which the body attacks its own tissues. Antibodies—our bodies' defenders against germs and other "foreign" substances in the blood—do the attacking. In the case of diabetes, antibodies attack and destroy the sensitive insulin-producing cells (beta cells) of the pancreas. For some reason, the body perceives these beta cells to be "foreign"—not made of its own familiar tissue.

But why would the body not recognize its own cells in the pancreas? That's a complicated question—and one that researchers will be working on for a long time. We do know quite a few things, however. The protein in cow's milk implicated by most researchers as a possible trigger for diabetes is called bovine serum albumin (BSA). Proteins such as BSA are made up of long strings of amino acids. It seems that BSA has a segment of 17 amino acids that resembles a segment on the surface of the beta cells in the pancreas.

However, when babies are born, their intestines aren't mature enough to properly digest certain foods. They can't break down proteins properly, and the walls of their intestines are too porous—they let large hunks of protein pass through into the bloodstream. That's not a good situation. The body may see these extra-large proteins as foreign objects and create antibodies to attack them, just as if they were invading bacteria. In the case of cow's milk, one of these proteins is BSA.

You can probably guess what researchers suspect may happen when antibodies are formed against BSA, given that BSA resembles certain areas on the beta cell in the pancreas. Like "friendly fire" in a war, the body may inadvertently destroy its own beta cells. Actually, this is a simplified version of the theory. Researchers believe that a complicated cascade of events—involving inflammatory processes and possible viral triggers—eventually result in pancreatic cell death.

What Is the Evidence for Cow's Milk As a Trigger for Type 1 Diabetes?

In 1992, an article published in the *New England Journal of Medicine* was the first to make a strong case for a cow's milk connection to diabetes.[2] The researchers reported a study conducted in Finland in which 142 newly diagnosed type 1 diabetic Finnish children were compared to 79 healthy children and 300 random adult blood donors. The researchers compared levels of antibodies to certain cow's milk proteins in the various groups. Although they found low levels of antibodies to BSA in some of the healthy children and adults, the levels in the diabetic children were an average of seven times higher! They did not find high levels of antibodies to other cow's milk proteins (casein and beta-lactoglobulin) in any of the groups.

Children fed cow's milk within the first 3 months of life appeared to be 1.4 times more likely to develop diabetes.

A French study found similar results: high levels of antibodies to BSA in 74.4% of newly diagnosed diabetics, but in only 5.5% of healthy controls.[3] These researchers also looked at children who had a potentially pre-diabetic condition identified by the presence of elevated antibodies to the beta cells, and found high levels of antibodies to BSA in 20% of these children.

The theory was intriguing enough for a "meta-analysis," which is a mathematical review that combines the results of all the studies that had already been done.

Putting everything together, children fed cow's milk within the first 3 months of life appeared to be 1.4 times more likely to develop diabetes.[4] Although not all studies have found a connection between cow's milk and diabetes,[5] the evidence on the whole appears to establish such a link.

Because of the evidence from these earlier studies, a truly large-scale study was launched in Europe called the Cow's Milk Avoidance Trial. Ten thousand infants who have siblings with type 1 diabetes are being given either a cow's milk–based formula or a non-cow's milk–based formula

The results of the study are still a few years away. However, it may be best to avoid giving your infant cow's milk at least during the first 6 months of life. The best option, if it is possible, is breastfeeding. Breastfeeding provides children with nature's best nutrition, boosts their immune systems against common childhood diseases, and may help prevent food allergies. If breastfeeding is not practical, another alternative is soy-based formula.

Is cow's milk appropriate for older children? The risk of cow's milk in diabetes may be limited primarily to babies under 6 months of age, when their intestines are most permeable to BSA proteins. If you do wish to keep an older child off milk, don't neglect to provide enough calcium through alternative sources, such as calcium-fortified orange juice, rice milk, soy milk, or daily calcium supplementation.

As an aside, evidence also shows that diets high in nitrates, found in smoked and pickled foods in particular, may also contribute to the development of type 1 diabetes.[6]

Niacinamide: Can Diabetes Be Prevented by Taking a Simple B Vitamin?

Besides breastfeeding young children, you may be able to reduce the risk of diabetes in another way. In the last 10 years, some exciting research has been conducted on the effect of niacinamide, a form of vitamin B$_3$. Provocative evidence suggests that niacinamide might be able to prevent diabetes in children at high risk.

A huge study conducted in New Zealand set out to determine whether niacinamide can prevent diabetes in school-age children.[7]

The results were fascinating and have several interesting implications. In this study, an enormous group of children—more than 20,000—were screened for ICA antibodies. It turned out that 185 of these children had detectable levels of ICA antibodies. About 170 of these children were then given niacinamide for 7 years (not all parents agreed to give their children niacinamide, or stay in the study for that long). About 10,000 other children were not screened, but they were followed to see whether they developed diabetes.

Provocative evidence suggests that niacinamide, a form of vitamin B$_3$, might be able to prevent diabetes in children at high risk.

The results were impressive. In the group where children were screened and given niacinamide when positive for ICA antibodies, the number of cases of diabetes was reduced by perhaps as much as 60%. These findings suggest that not only is niacinamide an effective treatment for preventing diabetes, but that ICA antibodies are a very effective screening tool. The statistics indicate that very few children without ICA-positive antibodies developed diabetes.

These results were so encouraging that in 1993, another large-scale trial called the European Nicotinamide Diabetes Intervention Trial was launched; it, too, is still in

Jonathan's Story

At age 15, Jonathan was admitted to the hospital for extreme lethargy. His doctor tested his blood sugar, which turned out to be 600. Diagnosed with type 1 diabetes, Jonathan was put on insulin and his condition stabilized, although his glucose was still higher than normal when he was discharged 4 days later.

My colleague, a naturopathic physician, saw Jonathan 2 days after his hospital discharge. Jonathan was extremely upset about the idea of taking insulin shots and his parents wanted to know whether there was any way to delay the inevitable. Admitting that he didn't know whether it would work, my colleague suggested that Jonathan take 3 g of niacinamide, 1,000 mcg chromium, and 20 mg vanadyl sulfate daily, while closely monitoring Jonathan's blood glucose levels. Everyone was happy when his glucose levels began to drop. Under the guidance of both his medical and naturopathic doctors, Jonathan gave himself less and less insulin, always keeping a close eye on his blood glucose. One week later, he was off all insulin, and maintaining normal blood

progress. Subjects are receiving either niacinamide (also called nicotinamide) or placebo.

A smaller trial, the Deutsche Nicotinamide Intervention Study, has been completed.[8] This study failed to find a significant protective effect of nicotinamide in people at especially high risk for developing diabetes. The two groups (nicotinamide and placebo) were observed for an average of 2.1 years. However, until the evidence comes in from other parts of the study, it is impossible to draw firm conclusions.

sugar. Jonathan remained totally off insulin for about 8 months. Then his blood sugar began to creep up, requiring small amounts of insulin to keep it normal. But he was more psychologically prepared by this time.

What Jonathan experienced over that 8 months was what doctors refer to as a "honeymoon period." Soon after a young person begins taking insulin after diagnosis of type 1 diabetes, it's fairly common for his or her pancreas to resume insulin production for a while. Would Jonathan have experienced an 8-month honeymoon period without the supplements? It's impossible to know, since honeymoon periods occasionally have been known to last for years.

It is vital to note that Jonathan was under the care of his medical doctor and his naturopathic physician during this time. In addition, he was closely monitoring his blood sugar at home. The importance of medical supervision for those taking high doses of supplements and adjusting insulin dosages can not be overemphasized.

Should You Give Your Child Niacinamide?

Suppose your child tests positive for ICA antibodies or has a history of diabetes in a parent or sibling. Before you rush out and start giving your child niacinamide, discuss the issue with your physician. Unlike breastfeeding, treatment with niacinamide may pose certain risks (see Safety Issues). Since the benefits are not yet established beyond doubt, these risks must be considered very seriously.

If your child already has developed diabetes, giving him or her niacinamide will probably not reverse the

disease, although some evidence suggests that it might
prolong the so-called honeymoon period when the body
can still make some insulin.[9–11]

How Does Niacinamide Prevent Diabetes?

We don't know for sure how niacinamide might help prevent diabetes, although we have some educated guesses.
Niacinamide seems to be able to interfere with certain enzymes that have the potential to indirectly destroy those
sensitive beta cells.

Dosage

The dosage of niacinamide used in many of the studies is
in the range of 25 mg/kg/day for children. There are 2.2
pounds in a kilogram, so a 40-pound child would get
around 450 mg daily. Some of the studies used somewhat
lower doses for children—in the range of 100 to 200 mg
daily. Adults have been prescribed as much as 2 to 3 g
daily.

Warning: Niacinamide should be distinguished from
niacin, a related vitamin that is used for lowering cholesterol. Because only the niacinamide form is believed to be
helpful in preventing diabetes, be sure to take this form.

Safety Issues

Niacinamide taken at a dose of several hundred milligrams daily generally causes no side effects. However,
some evidence indicates that high-dose niacinamide might
actually interfere with the action of insulin in healthy
people.[12] Future niacinamide trials should make sure to
look for this potential side effect. In the meantime, your
physician may wish to test your child for insulin sensitivity.

Furthermore, both niacin and niacinamide may cause
inflammation in the liver when taken at high doses. This is
another reason to make sure that a physician monitors your
child if you choose to use niacinamide for prevention.

The Future of Prevention of Type 1 Diabetes

Three large clinical trials are underway to determine whether type 1 diabetes can be prevented in people who are at risk but have not yet been diagnosed with the disease:

The Cow's Milk Avoidance Trial. This study, which involves infants who have a brother or sister with diabetes, randomly assigned participants to receive either a cow's milk-based formula or a non-dairy protein formula.

The European Nicotinamide Diabetes Intervention Trial. People at high risk for developing diabetes are receiving either niacinamide or placebo.

The Diabetes Prevention Trial—Type 1. This large study is examining the effects of giving low-dose insulin injections to people who are at risk for diabetes but do not yet have the disease. Some earlier studies suggested that such treatment may help prevent the disease from developing, perhaps by giving the pancreas a rest. Results of the larger study won't be in until the turn of the century . . . at least.

Depending on the results of these trials, large-scale screening of children for diabetes risk factors may be warranted. If such a practice becomes routine, it's conceivable that the incidence of this devastating illness could be significantly reduced.

A Word About Preventing Type 2 Diabetes

Type 2 diabetes is a different entity from type 1, so it makes sense that approaches to prevention are very different as well. Unlike type 1, prevention of type 2 diabetes involves lifestyle factors such as diet and exercise. Researchers also use different methods to determine who is at higher risk for each type of diabetes.

In the case of type 1 diabetes, researchers can test levels of the antibodies against the pancreas. Type 2 diabetes lacks these markers. Instead, many of the known risk factors for type 2 don't require a blood test to determine. They include obesity, a family history of the disease, and membership in certain ethnic groups—Native American, African-American, Hispanic, or Japanese-American.

About 85% of type 2 diabetics are either obese or have a past history of obesity. That means they're not just plump; they are seriously overweight. The causes of obesity vary. Some people may be obese because they eat too much fatty food or too many calories; or they may not be getting enough exercise to burn off the calories they eat. Some people seem to possess the kind of metabolism that can create fat even on a relatively low-calorie diet. It has also been suggested that some people may have an unidentified "fatness gene" that causes the body to store food to protect itself in case of famine. Whatever its cause, obesity can cause insulin to be less effective, resulting in elevated blood sugar. Losing weight can prevent the disease from occurring in the first place as well as actually "cure" the disease once it has manifested.

A group of researchers studied the eating patterns of Native Americans. Over the last 40 years, their eating patterns underwent a profound change. They changed from eating a diet based on whole, home-cooked foods and garden-grown vegetables to eating fast food on the run. The researchers found that their incidence of mortality from diabetes has risen 565% for men and a whopping 1,105% for women![13]

Even without a blood test, you can probably figure out to some extent whether you fall into a higher-than-average risk group for type 2 diabetes. Do you carry more weight than you should? (See chapter 1 for a discussion of "BMI"—the new way health professionals determine overweight.) Do you fall into one of the ethnic groups mentioned? Do you have a family history of the disease? If so, you may want to take some steps to protect yourself from developing type 2 diabetes.

Get More Exercise

Regular aerobic exercise is a wonderful way to lose weight, and losing weight is one of the best ways to protect yourself from type 2 diabetes if you tend toward obesity. Exercise can also lower blood sugar and improve cardiovascular functioning. If you've been sedentary or are over 40, check with your doctor before beginning a new exercise program. A strenuous new activity may unmask a hidden heart problem.

Eat a Healthy Diet

If you're at risk for type 2 diabetes because you are overweight, the best preventive approach may be to eat a healthy diet designed to trim your waistline. If you're not overweight but still at risk for type 2 diabetes, should you change your diet? It's not clear at this point whether eating specific foods will or will not prevent diabetes, although a recent study seems to indicate this might be true. Researchers found a possible role of dietary carotenes in the prevention of diabetes and insulin resistance. In particular, beta-carotene (found in high concentrations in yellow vegetables and fruits) and lycopene (especially high in tomatoes) were found to be lower in people with diabetes than in the general population. The researchers speculated these lower levels may contribute to diabetes and insulin resistance.[14] Please refer to chapter 2 for dietary controversies and recommendations.

In addition to the risk factors discussed above, scientists continue to look for screening techniques they can use to determine who is most at risk. In June 1996, the

American Diabetes Association announced a large new study: the Diabetes Prevention Program (DPP). The study is testing whether treating people who have impaired glucose tolerance will prevent the onset of type 2 diabetes. Four thousand people with impaired glucose metabolism have volunteered and will be followed for more than 4 years.[15] Some are receiving intensive lifestyle intervention with diet and exercise; others take oral diabetes drugs; and still others serve as a control group. Unfortunately, the study will not be looking at supplements such as chromium, which potentially could decrease insulin resistance much the same way some oral drugs do. (See chapter 3 for more information on chromium.)

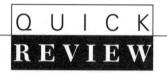

- Diabetes prevention in children known to be at special risk may be possible.
- If you have a parent, child, or sibling with type 1 diabetes, your risk of developing the disease is 10%.
- Risks approach 62% for children who have ICA antibodies.
- Preliminary research suggests that avoiding cow's milk for the first months of life reduces the risk of diabetes. A major study is now underway to determine whether this is true.
- In the meantime, if your child has a family history of type 1 diabetes, you may wish to avoid cow's milk—substituting breast milk or soy—in the first few months of life.
- Niacinamide, a form of vitamin B$_3$, may prevent diabetes in some individuals. A large study found niacinamide given to

high-risk schoolchildren cut the incidence of type 1 diabetes by more than half. Researchers are trying to confirm these findings in another large-scale study. Niacinamide should be distinguished from niacin, a related vitamin that is used for lowering cholesterol. Because only the niacinamide form is believed to be helpful in preventing diabetes, be sure you take this form.

- High-dose niacinamide for diabetes prevention should be used in children only under a doctor's supervision. It's best to first do blood testing to determine the child's risk level. The dosage of niacinamide used in many of the studies is in the range of 25 mg/kg/day for children. Some of the studies used somewhat lower doses for children—in the range of 100 to 200 mg daily.

- Currently three large clinical trials for the prevention of type 1 diabetes are underway: (1) the Cow's Milk Avoidance Trial, (2) the European Nicotinamide Diabetes Intervention Trial, and (3) the Diabetes Prevention Trial—Type 1. The latter is determining whether giving small doses of insulin to people at risk will prevent the development of the disease.

- Risk factors for type 2 diabetes include obesity, family history, and ethnicity.

- A study is presently underway to determine whether diet or drug therapy is more effective at preventing the disease in people with impaired glucose tolerance. Further study on natural supplements, such as chromium, for the prevention of type 2 diabetes seems warranted.

- Type 2 diabetes may be prevented by careful attention to diet and exercise. Often, loss of weight alone results in normalization of blood sugar.

Putting It All Together

F or your quick reference, this chapter contains a brief summary of key information contained in this book. Please refer to earlier chapters for more comprehensive information, including a detailed discussion of safety issues.

In this book I've given you an in-depth look at many natural remedies that may help control diabetes and prevent complications. They range from changes in dietary management to herbs and supplements shown to affect blood sugar and complications. You may feel overwhelmed at this point with so many approaches from which to choose. This summary will help you keep them all straight. You can use this chapter as a quick reference or share it with your doctor.

Natural Treatments for Blood Sugar Control

No supplements can replace insulin for people with type 1 diabetes. Even in type 2 diabetes, these supplements may only reduce rather than eliminate medication needs. Keep in mind that if these treatments are successful, you will need to adjust your medication to avoid hypoglycemia. For this reason, working closely with your physician is essential.

Considerable scientific evidence tells us that the mineral **chromium** can help keep blood sugar under control in both type 1 and type 2 diabetes. A typical dose of chromium is 200 to 600 mcg daily.

Other nutrients being researched include the minerals **vanadium** and **magnesium** and the **B vitamin biotin.**

A number of herbs may be helpful for aiding blood sugar control as well. Some scientific evidence supports the use of many of them, although none can be regarded as fully established. Those most commonly mentioned include **Gymnema, Momordica,** and **fenugreek.** *Gymnema sylvestre* is typically taken in doses of 400 to 600 mg daily of an extract standardized to contain 24% gymnemic acid. *Momordica charantia,* also called bitter melon, is best taken in the form of 2 ounces of fresh juice or 300 to 600 mg of the standardized extract daily. Fenugreek is recommended at a dosage of 25 to 50 g daily of the defatted seed powder, mixed with food or water. Other herbs with possible beneficial effects on blood sugar control include **garlic, onion, Pterocarpus, bilberry, *Coccinia indica*,** and **salt bush.**

Natural Treatments That May Help Prevent Diabetic Complications

Large-scale double-blind studies have shown that maintaining good control of blood sugar is key to preventing complications. In addition, a number of supplements and herbs may be helpful.

According to several double-blind studies, **lipoic acid** (200 mg 3 times daily with meals) can help reduce symptoms of diabetic neuropathy and is widely used for this purpose in Germany.

Double-blind studies have also found that GLA can reduce the symptoms of diabetic neuropathy if given several months to work. The usual dose is 3 to 4 g daily of **evening primrose oil. Borage** and **black currant oil** are also sometimes used because they are good sources of GLA.

Some evidence suggests that the following supplements may help prevent retinopathy: **bilberry, vitamin C,** and **vitamin E. Vitamin B_6** and **magnesium** may also be helpful.

Several supplements might help prevent cataracts, another eye disorder common among people with diabetes. These include **quercetin, vitamin C,** and **lipoic acid.**

Supplements which may help prevent heart and kidney disease in people with diabetes include **vitamin E, selenium, fish oils, ginkgo, vitamin C, magnesium, GLA, L-carnitine, oligomeric proanthocyanidins (grape seed extract),** and **garlic.**

Nutrient Deficiencies and Diabetes

Even if people with diabetes make sure to have a well-balanced diet, they tend to be deficient in several vitamins and minerals. Among the potential deficiencies are magnesium; several B vitamins; and vitamins A, C, and E. Other nutrients which may be deficient include coenzyme Q_{10} (CoQ_{10}) and essential fatty acids (EFAs).

Preventing Diabetes

Several studies suggest that avoiding cow's milk in early infancy may help prevent type 1 diabetes. For people whose blood tests suggest a high risk of type 1 diabetes, niacinamide supplements may also help prevent the disease.

Type 2 diabetes may be preventable by careful attention to diet and exercise. Often loss of weight results in normalization of blood sugar.

Diabetes is a challenge. Not only does it require constant attention to the details of diet, exercise, and blood sugar, it can also lead to complications that render life much more difficult. Many people who have diabetes are searching for new tools to improve their health. My hope is that if you have diabetes this book has given you new ideas that will help you better control your blood sugar and your life.

Notes

Chapter One

1. Saudek CD, et al., The Johns Hopkins guide to diabetes for today and tomorrow. Baltimore: The Johns Hopkins University Press, 22–29, 1997.

2. DCCT and Research Group. The effect of intensive treatment of diabetes on the development and progression of long-term complications in insulin-dependent diabetes mellitus. *New England Journal of Medicine* 329: 977–986, 1993.

Chapter Two

1. Elson DF and Meredith M. Therapy for type 2 diabetes mellitus. *Wisconsin Medical Journal* 97: 49–54, 1998.

Chapter Three

1. Anderson RA. Chromium metabolism and its role in disease processes in man. *Clinical Physiology and Biochemistry* 4: 31–41, 1986.

2. Anderson RA. Chromium as an essential nutrient for humans. *Regulatory Toxicology and Pharmacology* 26 (Pt.1 and 2): S35–S41, 1997.

3. Watts D. The nutritional relationships of chromium. *Journal of Orthopedic Medicine* 4: 17–23, 1989.

4. Anderson RA, et al. Elevated intakes of supplemental chromium improve glucose and insulin variables in individuals with type 2 diabetes. *Diabetes* 46: 1786–1791, 1997.

5. Ravina A and Slezak L. Chromium in the treatment of clinical diabetes mellitus. *Harefuah* 125(5–6): 142–145, 1993.

6. Ravina A, et al. Clinical use of the trace element chromium (III) in the treatment of diabetes mellitus. *Journal of Trace Elements in Medicine and Biology* 8: 183–190, 1985.

7. Evans GW. The effect of chromium picolinate on insulin-controlled parameters in humans. *International Journal of Biosocial and Medical Research* 11: 163–180, 1989.

8. Rabinowitz MB, et al. Effect of chromium and yeast supplements on carbohydrate and lipid metabolism in diabetic med. *Diabetes Care* 6: 319–327, 1983.

9. Hunt AE, et al. Effect of chromium supplementation on hair chromium and diabetic status. *Nutrition Research* 5: 131–140, 1985.

10. Anderson RA, et al. Lack of toxicity of chromium chloride and chromium picolinate in rats. *Journal of the American College of Nutrition* 16: 273–279, 1997.

11. Certulli J, et al. Chromium picolinate toxicity. *Annals of Pharmacotherapy* 32: 428–431, 1998.

12. Wasser WG, et al. Chronic renal failure after ingestion of over-the-counter chromium picolinate. *Annals of Internal Medicine* 126(5): 410, 1997.

13. Shamberger RJ. The insulin-like effects of vanadium. *Journal of Advances in Medicine* 9: 121–131, 1996.

14. Ramanadham S, et al. Oral vanadyl sulfate in treatment of diabetes mellitus in rats. *American Journal of Physiology* 257: 904–911, 1989.

15. Brichard SM, et al. Long-term improvement of glucose homeostasis by vanadate treatment in diabetic rats. *Endocrinology* 123: 2048–2053, 1988.

16. Kanthasamy A, et al. substitutes insulin role in chronic experimental diabetes. *Indian Journal of Experimental Biology* 26: 778–780, 1988.

17. Cohen N, et al. Oral vanadyl sulfate improves hepatic and peripheral insulin sensitivity in patients with non-insulin-dependent diabetes mellitus. *Journal of Clinical Investigation* 95: 2501–2509, 1995.

18. Halberstam M, et al. Oral vanadyl sulfate improves insulin sensitivity in NIDDM but not in obese nondiabetic subjects. *Diabetes* 45: 659–666, 1996.

19. Reddi A, et al. Biotin supplementation improves glucose and insulin tolerances in genetically diabetic KK mice. *Life Sciences* 42: 1323–1330, 1988.

20. Zhang H, et al. Biotin administration improves the impaired glucose tolerance of streptozotocin-induced diabetic Wistar rats. *Journal of Nutritional Science and Vitaminology* 43: 271–280, 1997.

21. Coggeshall JC, et al. Biotin status and plasma glucose in diabetics. *Annals of the New York Academy of Science* 447: 389–392, 1985.

22. Maebashi M, et al. Therapeutic evaluation of the effect of biotin on hyperglycemia in patients with non-insulin dependent diabetes mellitus. *Journal of Clinical Biochemistry and Nutrition* 14: 211–218, 1993.

23. Cleary JP. Vitamin B_3 in the treatment of diabetes mellitus. Case reports and review of the literature. *Journal of Nutrition and Medicine* 1: 217–225, 1990.

24. Lostroh AJ and Krahl ME. Magnesium, a second messenger for insulin: Ion transportation coupled to transport activity. *Advances in Enzyme Regulation* 12: 73–81, 1974.

25. Paolisso G, et al. Improved insulin response and action by chronic magnesium administration in aged NIDDM subjects. *Diabetes Care* 12: 265–269, 1989.

26. Garg A and Grundy SM. Nicotinic acid therapy for dyslipidemia in non-insulin-dependent diabetes mellitus. *Journal of the American Medical Association* 264: 723–726, 1990.

27. Faure P, et al. Zinc and insulin sensitivity. *Biological Trace Element Research* 32: 305–310, 1992.

28. Cunningham JJ, et al. Hyperzincuria in individuals with insulin-dependent diabetes mellitus: concurrent zinc status and the effects of high-dose zinc supplementation. *Metabolism* 43: 1558–1562, 1994.

29. Raz I, et. al. The influence of zinc supplementation on glucose homeostasis in NIDDM. *Diabetes Research II:* 73–79, 1989.

30. Cutler P. Desferrioxamine therapy in high-ferritin diabetes. *Diabetes* 38: 1207–1210, 1989.

Chapter Four

1. Shanmugasundarum ER, et al. Use of *Gymnema sylvestre* leaf in the control of blood glucose in insulin-dependent

diabetes mellitus. *Journal of Ethnopharmacology* 30: 281–294, 1990.

2. Baskaran K, et al. Antidiabetic effect of a leaf extract from *Gymnema sylvestre* in non-insulin-dependent diabetes mellitus patients. *Journal of Ethnopharmacology* 30: 295–305, 1990.

3. Prakash AO, et al. Effect of feeding *Gymnema sylvestre* leaves on blood glucose in beryllium nitrate treated rats. *Journal of Ethnopharmacology* 18: 143–146, 1986.

4. Shanmugasundarum ER, et al. Possible regeneration of the islets of Langerhans in streptozotocin-diabetic rats given *Gymnema sylvestre* leaf extracts. *Journal of Ethnopharmacology* 30: 265–279, 1990.

5. Shanmugasundarum KR, et al. Enzyme changes and glucose utilisation in diabetic rabbits: the effect of *Gymnema sylvestre*. R.Br. *Journal of Ethnopharmacology* 7: 205–234, 1983.

6. Shimizu K, et al. Suppression of glucose absorption by some fractions extracted from *Gymnema sylvestre* leaves. *Journal of Veterinary Medical Science* 59: 245–251, 1997.

7. Cunnick J and Takemoto D. Bitter melon (*Momordica charantia*). *Journal of Naturopathic Medicine* 4: 16–21, 1993.

8. Baldwa VS, et al. Clinical trial in patients with diabetes mellitus of an insulin-like compound obtained from plant sources. *Upsala Journal of Medical Sciences* 82: 39–41, 1977.

9. Welihinda J, et al. Effect of *Momordica charantia* on the glucose tolerance in maturity onset diabetes. *Journal of Ethnopharmacology* 17: 277–282, 1986.

10. Srivastava Y, et al. Antidiabetic and adaptogenic properties of *Momordica charantia* extract: An experimental and clinical evaluation. *Phytotherapy Research* 7: 285–289, 1993.

11. Akhtar MS. Trial of *Momordica charantia* Linn (Karela) powder in patients with maturity-onset diabetes. *Journal of the Pakistan Medical Association* 32: 106–107, 1982.

12. Leatherdale BA, et al. Improvement of glucose tolerance due to *Momordica charantia* (Karela). *British Medical Journal* 282: 1823–1824, 1981.

13. Sarkar S, et al. Demonstration of the hypoglycemic action of *Momordica charantia* in a validated animal model of diabetes. *Pharmacological Research* 33: 1–4, 1996.

14. Shibib BA, et al. Hypoglycaemic activity of *Coccinia indica* and *Momordica charantia* in diabetic rats: depression of the hepatic gluconeogenic enzymes glucose-6-phosphatase and fructose-1,6-bisphosphate and elevation of both liver and red-cell shunt enzyme glucose-6-phosphate dehydrogenase. *Biochemical Journal* 292(Pt 1): 267–270, 1993.

15. Ribes G, et al. Antidiabetic effects of subfractions from fenugreek seeds in diabetic dogs. *Proceedings of the Society for Experimental Biology and Medicine* 182: 159–166, 1986.

16. Sharma RD, et al. Effect of fenugreek seeds on blood glucose and serum lipids in type I diabetes. *European Journal of Clinical Nutrition* 44: 301–306, 1990.

17. Madar Z, et al. Glucose-lowering effect of fenugreek in non-insulin dependent diabetics. *European Journal of Clinical Nutrition* 42: 51–54, 1988.

18. Sharma RD, et al. Use of fenugreek seed powder in the management of non-insulin dependent diabetes mellitus. *Nutrition Research* 16: 1331–1339, 1996.

19. Ajabnoor MA and Tilmisany AK. Effect of *Trigonella foenum graecum* on blood glucose levels in normal and alloxan-diabetic mice. *Journal of Ethnopharmacology* 22: 45–49, 1988.

20. Madar Z. New sources of dietary fibre. *International Journal of Obesity and Related Metabolic Disorders* 11(Suppl. 1): 57–65, 1987.

21. Khan AK, et al. Treatment of diabetes mellitus with *Coccinia indica*. *British Medical Journal* 280: 1044, 1980.

22. Shibib BA, et al., 1993.

23. Flexible dose open trial of Vijayasar in cases of newly diagnosed non-insulin-dependent diabetes mellitus. Indian Council of Medical Research (ICMR), Collaborating Centres, New Delhi. *Indian Journal of Medical Research* 108: 24–29, 1998.

24. Manickam M, et al. Antihyperglycemic activity of phenolics from *Pterocarpus marsupium*. *Journal of Natural Products* 60: 609–610, 1997.

25. Ahmad F, et al. Insulin like activity in (-) epicatechin. *Acta Diabetologia Latina* 26: 291–300, 1989.

26. Chakravarthy BK, et al. Functional beta cell regeneration in the islets of the pancreas in alloxan induced diabetic rats by (-)-epicatechin. *Life Sciences* 31: 2693–2697, 1982.

27. Sheehan EW, et al. The lack of effectiveness of (-)-epicatechin against alloxan induced diabetes in Wistar rats. *Life Sciences* 33: 593–597, 1983.

28. Bone AJ, et al. Assessment of the antidiabetic activity of epicatechin in streptozotocin-diabetic and spontaneously diabetic BB/E rats. *Bioscience Reports* 5: 215–221, 1985.

29. Yaniv Z, et al. Plants used for the treatment of diabetes in Israel. *Journal of Ethno-pharmacology* 19(2): 145–151, 1987.

30. Stern E. Successful use of *Atriplex halimus* in the treatment of type II diabetic patients. A preliminary study. Zamenhoff Medical Center, Tel Aviv, 1989.

31. Earon G, et al. Successful us of *Atriplex hamilus* in the treatment of type 2 diabetic patients. Controlled clinical research report on the subject of Atriplex. Unpublished study conducted at the Hebrew Univeristy, Jerusalem, 1989.

32. Cignarella A, et al. Novel lipid-lowering properties of *Vaccinium myrtillus* L. leaves, a traditional antidiabetic treatment, in several models of rat dyslipidaemia: a comparison with ciprofibrate. *Thrombosis Research* 84: 311–322, 1996.

33. Teixeira CC, et al. The effect of *Syzygium cumini* (L.) skeels on post-prandial blood glucose levels in non-diabetic rats and rats with streptozotocin-induced diabetes mellitus. *Journal of Ethnopharmacology* 56: 209–213, 1997.

34. Bever BO and Zahnd GR. Plants with oral hypoglycemic action. *Quarterly Journal of Crude Drug Research* 17: 139–196, 1979.

35. Mathew PT and Augusti KT. Hypoglycaemic effects of onion, *Allium cepa* Linn. on diabetes mellitus—a preliminary report. *Indian Journal of Physiology and Pharmacology* 19: 213–217, 1975.

36. Rumessen JJ, et al. Fructans of Jerusalem artichokes: Intestinal transport, absorption, fermentation, and influence on blood glucose, insulin, and C-peptide responses in healthy subjects. *American Journal of Clinical Nutrition* 52: 675–681, 1990.

37. Silver AA and Krantz JC. The effect of the ingestion of bur-dock root on normal and diabetic individuals. A preliminary report. *Annals of Internal Medicine* 5: 274–284, 1931.

Chapter Five

1. Gabbay KH. The sorbitol pathway and the complications of diabetes. *New England Journal of Medicine* 288: 831–836, 1979.

2. Tomlinson DR, et al. Prevention of defects of axonal trans-port in experimental diabetes by aldose reductase inhibitors. *Drugs* 32(Suppl 2): S15–S18, 1986.

3. Nickander KK, et al. Alpha-lipoic acid: antioxidant potency against lipid peroxidation of neural tissues *in vitro* and im-plications for diabetic neuropathy. *Free Radical Biology and Medicine* 21: 631–639, 1996.

4. Mayes PA. The pentose phosphate pathway and other path-ways of hexose metabolism. In: Murray RK, Granner DK, Mayes PA, Rodwell VW, eds. Harper's biochemistry. 24th ed. Stamford, CT: Appleton & Lange, 214, 1988.

5. Greene DA. Sorbitol, myo-inositol and sodium-potassium ATPase in diabetic peripheral nerve. *Drugs* 32: S6–S14, 1986.

6. Kim J, et al. Normalization of Na(+)-K(+)-ATPase activity in isolated membrane fraction from sciatic nerves of streptozo-tocin-induced diabetic rats by myo-inositol supplementation *in vivo* or protein kinase C agonists *in vitro*. *Diabetes* 40: 558–567, 1991.

7. Nagamatsu M, et al. Lipoic acid improves nerve blood flow, reduces oxidative stress and improves distal nerve conduc-tion in experimental diabetic neuropathy. *Diabetes Care* 18: 1160–1167, 1995.

8. Kagan VE, et al. Dihydrolipoic acid—A universal antioxi-dant both in the membrane and in the aqueous phase. Re-duction of peroxyl, ascorbyl, and chromanoxyl radicals. *Biochemical Pharmacology* 44: 1637–1649, 1992.

9. Ziegler D, et al. Treatment of symptomatic diabetic neu-ropathy with the anti-oxidant alpha-lipoic acid. A 3-week multicentre randomized controlled trial (ALADIN Study). *Diabetologia* 38: 1425–1433, 1995.

10. Kahler W, et al. Diabetes mellitus—a free radical-associated disease. Results of adjuvant antioxidant supplementation. *Zeitschrift fuer die Gesamte Innere Medizin und Ihre Grenzgebiete* 48: 223–232, 1993.

11. Ziegler D, et al. Effects of treatment with the antioxidant alpha-lipoic acid on cardiac autonomic neuropathy in NIDDM patients. A 4-month randomized controlled multicentre trial (DEKAN Study). Deutsche Kardiale Autonome Neuropathie. *Diabetes Care* 20: 369–373, 1997.

12. Nickander KK, et al., 1996.

13. Kahler W, et al., 1993.

14. Ou P, et al. Activation of aldose reductase in rat lens and metal-ion chelation by aldose reductase inhibitors and lipoic acid. *Free Radical Research* 25: 337–346, 1996.

15. Nagamatsu M, et al., 1995.

16. Packer L, et al. Alpha-lipoic acid as a biological antioxidant. *Free Radical Biology and Medicine* 19: 227–250, 1995.

17. Gal EM. Reversal of selective toxicity of (-)-a-lipoic acid by thiamine in thiamine-deficient rats. *Nature* 207: 535, 1965.

18. Packer L, et al. 1995.

19. Keen H, et al. Treatment of diabetic neuropathy with gamma-linolenic acid. The Gamma-Linolenic Acid Multicenter Trial Group. *Diabetes Care* 16: 1309–1310, 1993.

20. Jamal GA and Carmichael H. The effect of gamma-linolenic acid on human diabetic peripheral neuropathy: a double-blind, placebo-controlled trial. *Diabetes Medicine* 7: 319–323, 1990.

21. Cameron NE, et al. Effects of alpha-lipoic acid on neurovascular function in diabetic rats. *Diabetologia* 41: 390–399, 1998.

22. Hounsom L, et al. A lipoic acid-gamma linolenic acid conjugate is effective against multiple indices of experimental diabetic neuropathy. *Diabetologia* 41: 839–843, 1998.

23. Cameron NE and Cotter MA. Potential therapeutic approaches to the treatment or prevention of diabetic neuropathy: evidence from experimental studies. *Diabetes Medicine* 10: 593–605, 1993.

24. Cameron NE and Cotter MA. Comparison of the effects of ascorbyl gamma-linolenic acid and gamma-linolenic acid in the correction of neurovascular deficits in diabetic rats. *Diabetologia* 39: 1047–1054, 1996.

25. Horrobin DF. Nutritional and medical importance of gamma-linolenic acid. *Prostaglandins and Lipid Research* 31: 163–194, 1992.

26. Horrobin DF, 1992.

27. Horrobin DF. Essential fatty acids in the management of impaired nerve function in diabetes. *Diabetes* 46(Suppl 2): S90–S93, 1997.

28. Horrobin DF, et al. Gamma-linolenic acid: An intermediate in essential fatty acid metabolism with potential as an ethical pharmaceutical and as a food. *Revue of Contemporary Pharmacotherapy* 1: 1–45, 1990.

29. Quatraro A, et al. Acetyl-L-carnitine for symptomatic diabetic neuropathy. *Diabetologia* 38: 123, 1995.

30. Onofrj M, et al. L-acetylcarnitine as a new therapeutic approach for peripheral neuropathies with pain. *International Journal of Clinical Pharmaceutical Research* 15: 9–15, 1995.

31. Lowitt S, et al. Acetyl-L-carnitine corrects the altered peripheral nerve function of experimental diabetes. *Metabolism* 44: 677–680, 1995.

32. Lowitt S, et al., 1995.

33. Spagnoli A, et al. Long-term acetyl-L-carnitine treatment in Alzheimer's disease. *Neurology* 41: 1726–1732, 1991.

34. Stracke H, et al. A benfotiamine-vitamin B combination in treatment of diabetic polyneuropathy. *Experimental and Clinical Endocrinology and Diabetes* 104: 311–316, 1996.

35. McCann VJ and Davis RE. Serum pyridoxal concentrations in patients with diabetic neuropathy. *Australian and New Zealand Journal of Medicine* 8: 259–261, 1978.

36. Rieder HP, et al. Vitamin status in diabetic neuropathy (thiamine, riboflavin, pyridoxine, cobalamin and tocopherol). *Zeitschrift fur Ernahrungswiss (Darmstadt)* 19: 1–13, 1980.

37. Levin ER, et al. The influence of pyridoxine in diabetic peripheral neuropathy. *Diabetes Care* 4: 606–609, 1981.

38. Khan MA, et al. Vitamin B_{12} deficiency and diabetic neuropathy. *Lancet* 2: 768–770, 1969.

39. Rieder HP, et al., 1980.

40. Ide H, et al. Clinical usefulness of intrathecal injection of methylcobalamin in patients with diabetic neuropathy. *Clinical Therapeutics* 9: 183–192, 1987.

41. Davidson S. The use of vitamin B_{12} in the treatment of diabetic neuropathy. *Journal of the Florida Medical Association* 15: 717–720, 1954.

42. Sancetta SM, et al. The use of vitamin B_{12} in the management of the neurological manifestations of diabetes mellitus, with notes on the administration of massive doses. *Annals of Internal Medicine* 35: 1028–1048, 1951.

43. Salway JG, et al. Effect of myo-inositol on peripheral-nerve function in diabetes. *Lancet* 2: 1282–1284, 1978.

44. Gregersen G, et al. Oral supplementation of myo-inositol: Effects on peripheral nerve function in human diabetics and on the concentration in plasma, erythrocytes, urine and muscle tissue in human diabetics and normals. *Acta Neurologica Scandinavian* 67: 164–172, 1983.

45. Shigeta Y, et al. Effect of pantethine treatment on vibratory perception in patients with diabetic neuropathy. *Journal of Vitaminology* 12: 299–302, 1966.

Chapter Six

1. Freitas JP, et al. Glycosylation and lipid peroxidation in skin and in plasma in diabetic patients (in French). *Comptes Rendus des Seances de la Societe de Biologie et de ses Filiales* 191: 837–843, 1997.

2. Kowlura R, et al. Abnormalities of retinal metabolism in diabetes or galactosemia. II. Comparison of gamma-glutamyl transpeptidase in retina and cerebral cortex, and effects of antioxidant therapy. *Current Eye Research* 13: 891–896, 1994.

3. Losada M and Alio JL. Malondialdehyde serum concentration in type 1 diabetic with and without retinopathy. *Documenta Ophthalmologica* 93: 223–229, 1996.

4. Lu M, et al. Advanced glycation end products increase retinal vascular endothelial growth factor expression. *Journal of Clinical Investigations* 101: 1219–1224, 1998.

5. Vaccaro O, et al. Moderate hyperhomocysteinaemia and retinopathy in insulin-dependent diabetes. *Lancet* 349: 1102–1103, 1997.

6. Hultberg B, et al. Increased levels of plasma homocysteine are associated with nephropathy, but not severe retinopathy in type 1 diabetes mellitus. *Scandinavian Journal of Clinical Laboratory Investigations* 51: 277–282, 1991.

7. DCCT group. Early worsening of diabetic retinopathy in the Diabetes Control and Complications Trial. *Archives of Ophthalmology* 116: 874–886, 1998.

8. UK Prospective Diabetes Study (UKPDS) Group. Intensive blood-glucose control with sulphonylureas or insulin compared with conventional treatment and risk of complications in patients with type 2 diabetes (UKPDS 33). *Lancet* 352: 854–865, 1998.

9. Sinclair AJ, et al. An investigation of the relationship between free radical activity and vitamin C metabolism in elderly diabetic subjects with retinopathy. *Gerontology* 38: 268–274, 1992.

10. Rema M, et al. Does oxidant stress play a role in diabetic retinopathy? *Indian Journal of Ophthalmology* 43: 17–21, 1995.

11. Ceriello A, et al. New insights on non-enzymatic glycosylation may lead to therapeutic approaches for the prevention of diabetic complications. *Diabetic Medicine* 9: 297–299, 1992.

12. Davie SJ, et al. Effect of vitamin C on glycosylation of protein. *Diabetes* 41: 167–173, 1992.

13. Cox BD and Butterfield WJ. Vitamin C supplements and diabetic cutaneous capillary fragility. *British Medical Journal* 3: 205, 1975.

14. Ali SM and Chakraborty SK. Role of plasma ascorbate in diabetic microangiopathy. *Bangladesh Medical Research Council Bulletin* 15: 47–59, 1989.

15. Cox BD and Butterfield WJ, 1975.

16. Gerster H. No contribution of ascorbic acid to renal calcium oxalate stones. *Annals of Nutrition and Metabolism* 41(5): 269–282, 1997.

17. Creter D, et al. Effect of vitamin E on platelet aggregation in diabetic retinopathy. *Acta Haematologica* 62: 74–77, 1979.

18. Rema M, et al., 1995.

19. Ceriello A, et al., 1992.

20. Schleicher ED, et al. Increased accumulation of the glycoxidation product N(epsilon)-(carboxymethyl)lysine in human tissues in diabetes and aging. *Journal of Clinical Investigations* 99: 457–468, 1997.

21. Kowlura R, et al., 1994.

22. Kunisaki M, et al. Prevention of diabetes-induced abnormal retinal blood flow by treatment with d-alpha-tocopherol. *Biofactors* 7: 55–67, 1998.

23. Creter D, et al., 1979.

24. Boniface R and Robert AM. Effect of anthocyanins on human connective tissue metabolism in the human. *Klinische Monatsblatter fur Augenheilkunde* 209: 368–372, 1996.

25. Detre Z, et al. Studies on vascular permeability in hypertension: action of anthocyanosides. *Clinical Physiological Biochemistry* 4: 143–149, 1986.

26. Scharrer A and Oher M. Anthocyanosides in the treatment of retinopathies. *Klinische Monatsblatter fur Augenheilkunde* 178: 386–389, 1981.

27. Lietti A, et al. Studies on *Vaccinium myrtillus* anthocyanosides. I. Vasoprotective and anti-inflammatory activity. *Arzneimittelforschung* 26: 829–832, 1976.

28. Lietti A and Forni G. Studies on *Vaccinium myrtillus* anthocyanosides. II. Aspects of anthocyanin pharmacokinetics in the rat. *Arzneimittelforschung* 26: 832–835, 1976.

29. Eandi M. Unpublished results. Cited in Morazzoni P, et al. *Vaccinium myrtillus Fitoterapia* 67: 3–29, 1996.

30. Lowitt S, et al. Acetyl-L-carnitine corrects electroretinographic deficits in experimental diabetes. *Diabetes* 42: 1115–1118, 1993.

31. Hotta N, et al. Effect of propionyl-L-carnitine on oscillatory potentials in electroretinogram in streptozotocin-diabetic rats. *European Journal of Pharmacology* 311: 199–206, 1996.

32. McNair P, et al. Hypomagnesemia, a risk factor in diabetic retinopathy. *Diabetes* 27: 1075–1077, 1978.

33. Ellis JM, et al. A deficiency of vitamin B_6 is a plausible molecular basis of the retinopathy of patients with diabetes mellitus. *Biochemical and Biophysical Research Communications* 179: 615–619, 1991.

34. Nakai N, et al. Aldose reductase inhibitors: flavonoids, alkaloids, acetophenones, benzophenones, and spirohydantoins of chroman. *Archives of Biochemistry and Biophysics* 239: 491–496, 1985.

35. Varma SD. Inhibition of aldose reductase by flavonoids: possible attenuation of diabetic complications. *Progress in Clinical and Biological Research* 213: 343–358, 1996.

36. Kador PF. Overview of the current attempts toward the medical treatment of cataract. *Ophthalmology* 90: 352–364, 1983.

37. Chaudrey PS, et al. Inhibition of human lens aldose reductase by flavonoids, sulindac and indomethacin. *Biochemical Pharmacology* 32: 1995–1998, 1983.

38. Varma SD, et al. Implications of aldose reductase in cataracts in human diabetes. *Investigations of Ophthalmology and Visual Science* 18: 237–241, 1979.

39. Varma SD, et al. Diabetic cataracts and flavonoids. *Science* 195: 205–206, 1997.

40. Leunberger PM. Diabetic cataract and flavonoids (first results). *Klinische Monatsblatter fur Augenheilkunde* 172: 460–462, 1978.

41. Varma SD, et al. Refractive change in alloxan diabetic rabbits. Control by flavonoids I. *Acta Ophthalmologica* 58: 748–759, 1980.

42. Ou P, et al., 1996.

43. Cunningham JJ, et al. Vitamin C: an aldose reductase inhibitor that normalizes erythrocyte sorbitol in insulin-dependent diabetes mellitus. *Journal of the American College of Nutrition* 13: 344–350, 1994.

44. Vinson JA, et al. *In vitro* and *in vivo* reduction of erythrocyte sorbitol by ascorbic acid. *Diabetes* 38: 1036–1041, 1989.

45. Aida K, et al. Isoliquiritigenin: a new aldose reductase inhibitor from glycyrrhizae radix. *Planta Medica* 56: 254–258, 1990.

Chapter Seven

1. Beaudeaux JL, et al. Enhanced susceptibility of low-density lipoprotein to *in vitro* oxidation in type I and type II diabetic patients. *Clinical Chimica Acta* 239: 131–141, 1995.

2. UK Prospective Diabetes Study (UKPDS) Group. Intensive blood-glucose control with sulphonylureas or insulin compared with conventional treatment and risk of complications in patients with type 2 diabetes (UKPDS 33). *Lancet* 352: 854–865, 1998.

3. Schleicher E, et al. Pathobiochemical aspects of diabetic nephropathy. *Klinische Wochenschrift* 66: 873–882, 1988.

4. Cohen MP, et al. Nonenzymatic glycosylation of glomerular basement membrane. *Renal Physiology* 4: 90–95, 1981.

5. Bostom AG, et al. Elevated fasting total plasma homocysteine levels and cadiovascular disease outcomes in maintenance dialysis patients. A prospective study. *Arteriosclerosis, Thrombosis, and Vascular Biology* 17: 2554–2558, 1997.

6. O'Brien SF, et al. Lipids, lipoproteins, antioxidants and glomerular and tubular dysfunction in type 1 diabetes. *Diabetes Research and Clinical Practice* 32: 81–90, 1996.

7. Jain SK, et al. Effect of modest vitamin E supplementation on blood glycated hemoglobin and triglyceride levels and red blood cell indices in type 1 diabetic patients. *Journal of the American College of Nutrition* 15: 458–461, 1996.

8. Onuma T, et al. Effect of vitamin E on plasma lipoprotein abnormalities in diabetic rats. *Diabetes Nutrition and Metabolism* 6: 135–138, 1993.

9. Fuller CJ, et al. RRR-alpha-tocopheryl acetate supplementation at pharmacologic doses decreases low-density-lipoprotein oxidative susceptibility but not protein glycation in patients with diabetes mellitus. *American Journal of Clinical Nutrition* 63: 753–759, 1996.

10. Reaven PD, et al. Effects of vitamin E on susceptibility of low-density lipoprotein and low-density lipoprotein subfractions to oxidation and on protein glycosylation in diabetes. *Diabetes Care* 18: 807–816, 1995.

11. Jenkins AJ, et al. LDL from patients with well-controlled IDDM is not more susceptible to *in vitro* oxidation. *Diabetes* 45: 762–767, 1996.

12. Colette C, et al. Platelet function in type I diabetes: effects of supplementation with large doses of vitamin E. *American Journal of Clinical Nutrition* 47: 256–261, 1988.

13. Gisinger C, et al. Effect of vitamin E supplementation on platelet thromboxane A2 production in type I diabetic patients. *Diabetes* 37: 1260–1264, 1988.

14. Dzhavad-zade MD, et al. Disorders of pulmonary hemodynamics in patients with diabetic nephroangiopathy and its correction with antioxidants. (in Russian) *Problemy Endokrinology (Moskow)* 38: 20–22, 1992.

15. Koya D, et al. Prevention of glomerular dysfunction in diabetic rats by treatment with d-alpha-tocopherol. *American Society of Nephrology* 8: 426–435, 1997.

16. Koya D, et al. D-alpha-tocopherol treatment prevents glomerular dysfunction in diabetic rats through inhibition of protein kinase C-diacylglycerol. *Biofactors* 7: 69–76, 1998.

17. Osterode W, et al. Nutritional antioxidants, red cell membrane fluidity and blood viscosity in type 1 (insulin dependent) diabetes mellitus. *Diabetes Medicine* 13: 1044–1050, 1996.

18. Douilet C, et al. A selenium supplement associated or not with vitamin E delays early renal lesions in experimental diabetes in rats. *Proceedings of the Society for Experimental Biology and Medicine* 211: 323–331, 1996.

19. Friday KE, et al. Omega-3 fatty acid supplementation has discordant effects on plasma glucose and lipoproteins in type II diabetes. *Diabetes* 36(Suppl. 1): 12A, 1987.

20. Jensen T, et al. Partial normalization by dietary cod-liver oil of increased microvascular albumin leakage in patients with insulin-dependent diabetes and albuminuria. *New England Journal of Medicine* 321: 1572–1577, 1989.

21. Goh YK, et al. Effect of omega 3 fatty acid on plasma lipids, cholesterol and lipoprotein fatty acid content in NIDDM patients. *Diabetologia* 40: 45–52, 1997.

22. Jones DB, et al. Indirect evidence of impairment of platelet desaturase enzymes in diabetes mellitus. *Hormone and Metabolic Research* 18: 341–344, 1986.

23. Kamada T, et al. Dietary sardine oil increases erythrocyte membrane fluidity in diabetic patients. *Diabetes* 35: 604–611, 1986.

24. Haines AP, et al. Effects of fish oil supplement on platelet function, haemostatic variables and albuminuria in insulin-dependent diabetics. *Thrombosis Research* 43: 643–655, 1986.

25. Laganiere S and Fernandes G. High peroxidizability of sub-cellular membrane induced by high fish oil diet is reversed by vitamin E. *Clinical Research* 35: A565, 1987.

26. Houtsmuller AJ, et al. Favourable influences of linoleic acid on the progression of diabetic micro- and macroangiopathy. *Nutrition and Metabolism* 24(Suppl 1): 105–118, 1980.

27. Ginter E, et al. Hypocholesterolemic effect of ascorbic acid in maturity-onset diabetes mellitus. *International Journal for Vitamin and Nutrition Research* 48: 368–373, 1978.

28. Sakurauchi Y, et al. Effects of L-carnitine supplementation on muscular symptoms in hemodialyzed patients. *American Journal of Kidney Disease* 32: 258–264, 1998.

29. Sloan RS, et al. Quality of life during and between hemodialysis treatments: role of L-carnitine supplementation. *American Journal of Kidney Diseases* 32: 265–272, 1998.

30. Bazzato G, et al. Myasthenia-like syndrome after DL- but not L-carnitine. *Lancet* 1: 1209, 1981.

31. Lagrue G, et al. A study of the effects of procyanidol oligomers on capillary resistance in hypertension and in certain nephropathies. *Semaine des Hopitaux Paris* 57: 1399–1401, 1981.

32. Werbach MR and Murray MT. Botanical influences on illness: a sourcebook of clinical research. Tarzana, CA: Third Line Press, 28, 1994.

33. Franconi F, et al. Plasma and platelet taurine are reduced in subjects with insulin-dependent diabetes mellitus: effects of taurine supplementations. *American Journal of Clinical Nutrition* 61: 1115–1119, 1995.

34. Trachtman H, et al. Taurine ameliorates chronic strepto-zocin-induced diabetic nephropathy in rats. *American Journal of Physiology* 269: F429–F438, 1995.

35. Elamin A and Tuvemo T. Magnesium and insulin-dependent diabetes mellitus. *Diabetes Research and Clinical Practice* 10: 203–209, 1990.

Chapter Eight

1. Rieder HP, et al., 1980.

2. Elamin A and Tuvemo T. Magnesium and insulin-dependent diabetes mellitus. *Diabetes Research and Clinical Practice* 10: 203–209, 1990.

3. Durlach J and Collery P. Magnesium and potassium in diabetes and carbohydrate metabolism. Review of the present status and recent results. *Magnesium* 3: 315–323, 1984.

4. Sjogren A, et al. Magnesium, potassium and zinc deficiency in subjects with type II diabetes mellitus. *Acta Medica Scandinavian* 224: 461–466, 1988.

5. McNair P, et al. Hypomagnesemia, a risk factor in diabetic retinopathy. *Diabetes* 27: 1075–1077, 1978.

6. Cunningham J. Reduced mononuclear leukocyte ascorbic acid content in adults with insulin-dependent diabetes mellitus consuming adequate dietary vitamin C. *Metabolism* 40: 146–149, 1991.

7. Zabrowski EJ and Bhatnagar PK. Urinary excretion pattern of ascorbic acid in streptozotocin diabetic and insulin treated rats. *Pharmacological Research Communications* 11: 95–103, 1979.

8. Som S, et al. Ascorbic acid metabolism in diabetes. *Metabolism* 30: 572–577, 1981.

9. Padh H, et al. Glucose inhibits cellular ascorbic acid uptake by fibroblasts *in vitro*. *Cell Biology International Report* 9: 531–538, 1985.

10. Hodges R. Drug-nutrient interactions. In: Nutrition in medical practice. Philadelphia: W.B. Saunders, 323–331, 1980.

11. Basu TK, et al. Serum vitamin A and retinol-binding protein in patients with insulin-dependent diabetes mellitus. *American Journal of Clinical Nutrition* 50: 329–331, 1989.

12. Wako Y, et al. Vitamin A transport in plasma of diabetic patients. *Tohoku Journal of Experimental Medicine* 149: 133–143, 1986.

13. Lubin B and Machlin L. Biological aspects of vitamin E. *Annals of the New York Academy of Science* 393, 1982.

14. Basu TK, et al., 1989.

15. Koutsikos D, et al. Biotin for diabetic peripheral neuropathy. *Biomedicine and Pharmacotherapy* 44: 511–514, 1990.

16. Kosenko LG. *Klinical Medizine* 42: 113, 1964.

17. Ditzel J. Oxygen transport impairment in diabetes. *Diabetes* 25: 832–838, 1976.

18. Sjogren A, et al., 1988.

19. Pai LH and Prasad A. Cellular zinc in patients with diabetes mellitus. *Nutrition Research* 8: 889–898, 1988.

20. Mateo MC, et al. Serum zinc, copper and insulin in diabetes mellitus. *Biomedicine* 29: 56–58, 1978.

21. Sjogren A, et al., 1988.

22. Durlach J and Collery P, 1984.

23. Perez GO, et al. Potassium homeostasis in chronic diabetes mellitus. *Archives of Internal Medicine* 137: 1018–1022, 1977.

24. Smoller S, et al. Blunted kaliuresis after an acute oral potassium load in diabetes mellitus. *American Journal of the Medical Sciences* 295: 114–121, 1988.

25. Mercuri O, et al. Depression of microsomal desaturation of linoleic to gamma-linolenic acid in the alloxan-diabetic rat. *Biochimie et Biophysica Acta* 116: 409–411, 1966.

26. Jones DB, et al., 1986.

27. Kishi T, et al. Bioenergetics in clinical medicine. XI. Studies on coenzyme Q and diabetes mellitus. *Journal of Medicine* 7: 307–321, 1976.

Chapter Nine

1. Bingley PJ, et al. Combined analysis of autoantibodies improves prediction of IDDM in islet cell antibody-positive relatives. *Diabetes* 43: 1304–1310, 1994.

2. Karjalainen J, et al. A bovine albumin peptide as a possible trigger of insulin-dependent diabetes. *New England Journal of Medicine* 327: 302–307, 1992.

3. Levy-Marchal C, et al. Antibodies against bovine albumin and other diabetic markers in French children. *Diabetes Care* 18: 1089–1094, 1995.

4. Gerstein HC. Cow's milk exposure and type 1 diabetes mellitus. *Diabetes Care* 17: 13–19, 1994.

5. Norris JM, et al. Lack of association between early exposure to cow's milk protein and beta-cell autoimmunity. Diabetes Autoimmunity Study in the Young (DAISY). *Journal of the American Medical Association* 276: 609–614, 1996.

6. Dahlquist GG, et al. Dietary factors and the risk of developing insulin dependent diabetes in childhood. *British Medical Journal* 300: 1302–1306, 1990.

7. Elliott RB, et al. A population based strategy to prevent insulin-dependent diabetes using nicotinamide. *Journal of Pediatric Endocrinology and Metabolism* 9: 501–509, 1996.

8. Lampeter EF, et al. The Deutsche Nicotinamide Intervention Study: an attempt to prevent type 1 diabetes. DENIS Group. *Diabetes* 47: 980–984, 1998.

9. Pozzilli P, et al. Meta-analysis of nicotinamide treatment in patients with recent-onset IDDM. The Nicotinamide Trialists. *Diabetes Care* 19: 1357–1363, 1996.

10. Pozzilli P, et al. Double blind trial of nicotinamide in recent-onset IDDM (the IMDIAB III study). *Diabetologia* 38: 848–852, 1995.

11. Vague P, et al. Effect of nicotinamide treatment on the residual insulin secretion in type 1 (insulin-dependent) patients. *Diabetologia* 32: 316–321, 1989.

12. Greenbaum CJ, et al. Nicotinamide's effect on glucose metabolism in subjects at risk for IDDM. *Diabetes* 45: 1631–1634, 1996.

13. Gilliland FD, et al. Temporal trends in diabetes mortality among American Indians and Hispanics in New Mexico: birth cohort and period effects. *American Journal of Epidemiology* 145: 422–431, 1997.

14. Ford ES, et al. Diabetes mellitus and serum carotenoids: findings from the Third National Health and Nutrition Examination Survey. *American Journal of Epidemiology* 149: 168–176, 1999.

15. Linday LA. Trivalent chromium and the diabetes prevention program. *Medical Hypotheses* 49: 47–49, 1997.

Index

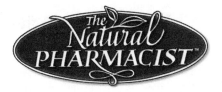

About the Author

Kathleen Head, N.D., is a 1985 graduate of the National College of Naturopathic Medicine in Portland, Oregon. Following graduation, she practiced naturopathic medicine for 11 years in San Diego. In the spring of 1997 she moved to Sandpoint, Idaho, to take a position as technical adviser for Thorne Research, a nutritional supplement, education, and research company. She is also senior editor for the peer-reviewed, MEDLINE-indexed journal, *Alternative Medicine Review.*

She has served as Director of Educational Affairs for the American Association of Naturopathic Physicians since 1990. Her articles on a variety of health topics have appeared widely in both popular and professional publications. She took a special interest in diabetes because of personal friends and a favorite cat with the disease, lecturing and writing on the topic for both lay and professional audiences.

About the Series Editors

Steven Bratman, M.D., medical director of Prima Health, h[as] many years of experience in the alternative medicine field. [A] graduate of the University of California at Davis, Medical School, [he] has also trained in herbology, nutrition, Chinese medicine, and oth[er] alternative therapies, and has worked closely with a wide variety [of] alternative practitioners. He is the author of *The Natur[al] Pharmacist: Your Complete Guide to Herbs* (Prima), *The Natur[al] Pharmacist: Your Complete Guide to Illnesses and Their Natur[al] Remedies* (Prima), *The Natural Pharmacist Guide to St. John's W[ort] and Depression* (Prima), *The Alternative Medicine Ratings Gui[de]* (Prima), and *The Alternative Medicine Sourcebook* (Lowell Hous[e])

David J. Kroll, Ph.D., is a professor of pharmacology and toxicolo[gy] at the University of Colorado School of Pharmacy and a consulta[nt] for pharmacists, physicians, and alternative practitioners on t[he] indications and cautions for herbal medicine use. A graduate of bo[th] the University of Florida and the Philadelphia College of Pharma[cy] and Science, Dr. Kroll has lectured widely and has published artic[les] in a number of medical journals, abstracts, and newsletters.